Advance Praise for
The Happiest Baby Guide to Great Sleep

"Dr. Karp is a parenting hero! His *Happiest Baby Guide to Great Sleep* would have helped tremendously when I was an exhausted new mom. It's a must-have resource for all families."
— JANE HONIKMAN, M.S., FOUNDER OF POSTPARTUM SUPPORT INTERNATIONAL

"Sleep deprivation often pushes moms into postpartum depression. Dr. Karp's fabulous new book is at the top of my list to help all new parents get the sleep they need to stay healthy and enjoy this precious time of life."
— LUCY PURYEAR, M.D., MEDICAL DIRECTOR OF THE WOMEN'S PLACE: CENTER FOR REPRODUCTIVE PSYCHIATRY, TEXAS CHILDREN'S HOSPITAL

"Amazing! Dr. Karp has done it again! With wit and wisdom he reveals the simple steps to get precious extra hours of rest. This remarkable book will have your babies and toddlers sleeping in no time!"
— RONI COHEN LEIDERMAN, PH.D., DEAN OF MAILMAN SEGAL CENTER FOR HUMAN DEVELOPMENT, NOVA SOUTHEASTERN UNIVERSITY

"Mixing good science—with a welcome dose of humor—this once-in-a-generation sleep book will strengthen your skills and lower your stress."
— JETTA BERNIER, EXECUTIVE DIRECTOR OF MASSACHUSETTS CITIZENS FOR CHILDREN

"When your little child sleeps well . . . life just seems happier. Dr. Karp's unique and gentle ideas may be exactly what you've been dreaming of!"
— DIANE DEBROVNER, DEPUTY EDITOR AT PARENTS MAGAZINE

"Once again, Dr. Karp saves parent sanity (and rescues relationships). With his trademark smart, fast-acting advice, he'll help your child—and you—sleep better and longer!"

—Kyle Pruett, M.D., professor at Yale School of Medicine and coauthor of Partnership Parenting

"Dr. Karp's white noise advice is incredibly helpful for boosting sleep. I recommend it to my patients . . . and even use it with my own children!"

—Ian Paul, M.D., professor of pediatrics and public health, Penn State College of Medicine

"What a gift! Dr. Karp (once again) makes things so easy. You'll reconnect with the miracle of sleep faster than you can imagine . . . and you'll be the dad—and husband—you really want to be. It works!"

—Matt Goldman, cofounder of Blue Man Group and Blue School

"Finally, everything you need to know about sleep is all in one book! The Happiest Baby Guide to Great Sleep shows how to get a good night's sleep . . . without all the tears. It's a must-read for sleep-deprived parents!"

—Jennifer Shu, M.D., pediatrician and coauthor of Heading Home with Your Newborn: From Birth to Reality

"Dr. Karp rescues weary parents with great ideas that flip conventional wisdom right on its head! His fresh insights will help turn your bedtime screamer . . . into a champion sleeper."

—Harold Koplewicz, M.D., founder and president of Child Mind Institute

The Happiest Baby
Guide to Great Sleep

The Happiest Baby Guide to Great Sleep

Simple Solutions for Kids from Birth to 5 Years

HARVEY KARP, M.D.

wm

WILLIAM MORROW
An Imprint of HarperCollins*Publishers*

This book is designed to give information on various medical conditions, treatments and procedures for your personal knowledge and to help you be a more informed consumer of medical and health services. It is not intended to be complete or exhaustive, nor is it a substitute for the advice of your physician. You should seek medical care promptly for any specific medical condition or problem your child may have. Under no circumstances should medication of any kind be administered to your child without first checking with your physician.

All efforts have been made to ensure the accuracy of the information contained in this book as of the date published. The author and the publisher expressly disclaim responsibility for any adverse effects arising from the use or application of the information contained herein.

THE HAPPIEST BABY GUIDE TO GREAT SLEEP. Copyright © 2012 by The Happiest Baby, Inc. All rights reserved. Printed in the United States of America. No part of this book may be used or reproduced in any manner whatsoever without written permission except in the case of brief quotations embodied in critical articles and reviews. For information address HarperCollins Publishers, 10 East 53rd Street, New York, NY 10022.

HarperCollins books may be purchased for educational, business, or sales promotional use. For information please write: Special Markets Department, HarperCollins Publishers, 10 East 53rd Street, New York, NY 10022.

Designed by Richard Oriolo

Library of Congress Cataloging-in-Publication Data has been applied for.

ISBN 978-0-06-211331-3

12 13 14 15 16   OV/RRD   10 9 8 7 6 5 4 3

To the millions of great parents who pray for just . . . a little more sleep.

Your goal is truly within reach.

Contents

PART 3 | 201

Sleep Solutions in the Toddler and Preschool Years: One to Five Years

PART 4 | 301

Tips to Create Happy Naps and to Handle Special Situations

Acknowledgments

The only thing worth stealing is a kiss from a sleeping child.

—JOE HOULDSWORTH

While sleep is certainly a solitary endeavor, writing a book requires a gaggle of family, friends, and colleagues for inspiration and encouragement.

My deep gratitude to my soul mate, wife, and best friend, Nina. Thank you my sweetheart! Your constant love, steady support, wise advice, and great patience during my nights and weeks away meant more to me than I can tell you. My reward at the end of each day—*you*—truly made this book possible. (And, thank you Lexi for your love and enthusiasm.)

To my parents, Sophie and Joe, I can never thank you enough for giving me the education that has carried me like a ship through the sunsets and storms of my life.

Thanks to my dear friends Laurie David and Bart Thorpe for your support and inexhaustible passion for all that you do to make the world a better place (one plant and one planet at a time), and to Maja and Dimitri Vukcevic for all your friendship.

A salute to the scores of Starbucks and Coffee Beans across the west side of Los Angeles that served as my white noise filled, nomadic office.

A huge thanks to my Happiest Baby team!

To Kristin Moss for your creative mind and always positive attitude; to Neal Tabachnick for your persistence and good counsel; and to Marija Sipka, Emily Weese, Shaena Cushman, Louise Teeter, and Eva Glettner for your hard work and keeping our important mission alive even during my long hours away.

And to the thousands of Happiest Baby educators across America and around the world for your faith in my work and for your dedicated service to so many families in need.

A heartfelt appreciation to the enormously wise and talented Lisa Sharkey at HarperCollins. Thank you for your friendship and compassion and for your confidence in my work. And, a salute goes to your extraordinary sister, Tina Sharkey, and to her son, Charlie Goldstein! Charlie, like the siren's call, your colicky cries pulled me into the lucky company of your incredible mom and aunt.

I owe a debt of gratitude to the rest of my HarperCollins team, as well, including most especially, Amy Bendell (my skillful and patient editor) and Shelby Meizlik. You have worked hard to get this project onto the launching pad and ready for blast-off.

Thanks to my gifted mentor, Arthur Parmelee, and all the other great pediatricians and sleep experts from whom I have had the honor to learn. And, to my weekly brain group colleagues: Namhee Lee, Hans Miller, John Schumann, and Leon Sones for your love of knowledge and constant inspiration.

My deep bow of appreciation goes to all my friends and colleagues who so generously gave of their time to review this book and donate their comments, including Arianna Huffington, Agapi

Stassinopolous, Jane Honikman, Jetta Bernier, Matt Goldman and Drs. Gary Freed, John Harrington, Fran Kaufman, Harold Koplewicz, Roni Leiderman, Ian Paul, Kyle Pruett, Lucy Puryear, Harley Rotbart, Jennifer Shu, Alison Blakely, Diane Debrovner, and Steve Shelov.

Finally, my deepest gratitude goes to the thousands of children and parents I cared for during my thirty years of practice. And to the families who allowed me to observe and film their little ones and to all those who reached out over the years through phone calls, e-mails, and letters. Thank you for opening your hearts and inviting me into your lives. It has been one of the greatest privileges of my life to be a confidant in your joys and struggles. I am a very satisfied doctor if I have helped some of you get more sleep . . . feel more skilled . . . and raise healthier, happier children. Your belief in me and trust in my work has been my greatest reward!

The Happiest Baby
Guide to Great Sleep

Introduction

When children are young, you get no sleep.
When they're old, you get no rest.

—FOLK SAYING

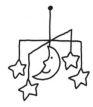

Does your baby melt your heart with love when you rock her to sleep . . . and then drive you totally insane for the rest of the night? Does your home become a battleground every night, as your tot flails and cries "No, no, no!" when it's time for *bed?*

Being a parent is the most wonderful experience you'll ever have. But having a child who is a bad sleeper hits you with a huge double whammy:

You feel like you're getting a big, fat D in Mommy-ing (or Daddy-ing).

Plus you're utterly exhausted.

Ahhh . . . sleep!!

If you're like most new moms, a good night's sleep shimmers

in your weary mind like a mirage in the desert. No wonder sleep struggles are the number one behavioral grumble of parents.

And it's not just about babies. A third of toddlers fight bedtime and half still get up once a night (one in ten wakes two times a night . . . or more!). No wonder a 2004 National Sleep Foundation poll found that millions of parents get less than six hours of sleep a night (one in five of those with infants and one in eight with tots and preschoolers).

Bone-weary parents often fall prey to overeating, quarreling, accidents, illness, anxiety, and even depression. And, like a rock thrown in a lake, exhaustion can trigger wave after wave of worry:

- **"Am I creating bad habits?"**
- **"Will 'crying it out' scar my baby emotionally?"**
- **"Should she be on a schedule?"**
- **"Will this ever stop?"**

Today's new parents have little experience with babies—amazingly, many have never even *touched* a newborn in their lives! So they seek answers from the piles of sleep manuals on bookstore shelves. (Over the past twenty years, more sleep manuals have come and gone than any other type of parenting book.)

Yet these guides often *misguide* parents, and make things even more confusing:

- **"Hold your baby . . . but don't spoil her!"**
- **"Swaddle your baby . . . but don't create a dependency!"**
- **"Love your baby . . . but shut the door and let her cry herself to sleep!"**

So it's no surprise that rookie parents flip-flop between feeling like major-league pros (on good days) and bumbling boobs (on those other days). And, on top of all this, most parents today have lost the strong support system that helped their great-grandparents manage: big, supportive families; close neighbors; and teenage girls down the street eager to babysit.

However, you can be reassured to know that billions of parents—stretching all the way back to the beginning of time—have successfully conquered these hurdles, which means that you can, too.

And that leads me to the best news of all: a few simple ideas—weaving together ancient wisdom and breakthrough science—can help you solve most of your child's sleep struggles in less than a week. (Or better yet, *prevent* them even before they happen!)

Sound too good to be true? I've heard that before. . . .

Parents and even many doctors were a bit skeptical when I introduced *The Happiest Baby* DVD and book a decade ago. But those very simple ideas have now helped millions of parents around the world calm their fussy babies—even most colicky ones—in minutes or less!

Likewise, the unexpected innovations in my DVD and book, *The Happiest Toddler,* surprised many by answering a problem that had vexed parents for centuries: Why are toddlers so unreasonable? Suddenly, parents had new ways to stop most tantrums fast and to help even easy tots become more patient and cooperative, in just days!

After thirty years of caring for thousands of babies I was so fortunate to uncover practical solutions to common problems . . . that work unexpectedly well and fast. And now, I am thrilled to offer you some simple—but surprising—steps to help your infant or young child sleep beautifully all through the night.

Times Change: A Goal and a Promise

It sounds almost unbelievable, but sixty years ago, few American moms nursed their babies. After tens of thousands of years of every single mother feeding her baby at the breast, women in our country almost lost this life-sustaining skill.

It took millions of dollars, decades of effort, and a nationwide education campaign to debunk the myth that factory-made formula was better than breast milk. But the effort was well worth it. Today, women across the country are confidently breast-feeding their babies. As a result, their children are healthier . . . and mothers are, too.

Now that we've popped the *formula-is-better-than-breast-milk* myth, my goal is to shatter another set of myths—sleep myths—that have confused and misled exhausted parents for centuries. For example:

- **Babies need to sleep in total quiet . . . Wrong!**
- **Rice cereal boosts an infant's sleep . . . Wrong!**
- **All infants sleep longer after three months of age . . . Wrong!**
- **Stomach gas and cramps cause babies to be wakeful and fussy . . . Wrong!**
- **Crying it out is the best way to sleep train a child . . . Wrong!**

My goal is to replace these mistaken ideas with new insights to quickly improve your child's sleeping . . . the *Happiest Baby* way. You'll discover:

- **Why you can't spoil your little baby.**
- **How to add an hour—or more—to your infant's sleep.**
- **Why waking sleeping babies actually boosts their sleep.**
- **Why white noise works sleepy-time magic at any age.**
- **Why your child's bedtime really starts . . . in the morning.**
- **Which bedtime routines work the best.**
- **A new, no-tears way to sleep train your tot . . . called *twinkle interruptus*.**

And here's my promise: your child's sleep problems can be prevented or solved—quickly and lovingly—probably with little or no "crying it out." Thousands of parents have gotten more sleep with the methods you're about to learn and I'm confident you will, too.

Parents joke that babies should come with instructions. Well, now they do! My dream is that these "instructions" will create a world where stories about sleepless babies and exhausted parents will only be found in history books and fairy tales. And I truly believe that these simple ideas will help you to have the happiest sleeper on your block!

The *Happiest Baby* Way— How to Use This Book

If you've read the *Happiest Baby* and *Happiest Toddler* books, you'll recognize some old favorite techniques . . . but this time, you'll learn how to adapt these techniques specifically for sleep. I'll identify these *Happiest Baby* way ideas and tips in a review section at the end of each chapter and I'll highlight my new sleep ideas in special sections, so you can find them more easily.

Also, as you go through the book, you may spot some information mentioned more than once. That's because, after you read the first chapter on the basics of sleep, you'll probably want to jump right to the section that best fits your child's age—and so I repeated a few key points so you don't have to keep going back in the book to find them.

## CHAPTER ONE

The Science of Sleep: Understanding the Beautiful, Deep Ocean of Slumber

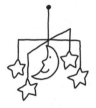

KEY POINTS:

★ **Sleep restores energy, boosts thinking, organizes memories, strengthens immunity, helps us lose weight, and so much more.**

★ **Sleep deprivation clouds our judgment, depresses our mood, and can lead to bad decisions, car accidents, heart disease . . . even cancer.**

★ **Each day is organized around Nature's cues— telling us to wake with the sun and fall asleep after dark. This circadian rhythm is directed by** the brain's release of a special sleep hormone (melatonin).

★ Sleep is made up of cycles of rapid eye movement sleep, or REM (the time of dreams and memory storage), and non-REM, restful sleep, which alternate over and over through the night.

★ Kids wake more often because they have shorter sleep cycles than adults (sixty versus ninety minutes).

★ Infants have up to five times more REM sleep, which lets them file away in their memories the flood of new things things they learn every day!

Every night I go abroad,
afar into the land of Nod . . .
—ROBERT LOUIS STEVENSON

The Dark Side of the Moon: What Happens When We Sleep?

If you're like most of the tired parents I meet every day, I'm guessing you don't really want a science lesson right now. Instead, you're saying: "Please, just tell me what to do!"

So feel free to jump ahead if you want. But many people find that a few facts about this wondrous state—sleep—helps put the advice in the rest of the book into perspective.

So let's take a quick look at what sleep really is.

The Facts—and Myths—About Sleep

Sleep is a contradiction! We spend a third of our lives in it, yet it seems as distant and as foreign as the depths of the ocean.

Over the past thirty years, sleep has come under the scrutiny of many brilliant scientists. And thanks to their research, the things we're learning about this misty frontier are dispelling centuries' worth of misconceptions. For example:

MYTH 1: *When you're asleep, you're unconscious.*

FACT: Sleep is not coma. We can hear the phone ring or the alarm clock buzz. Some folks even talk and walk in their sleep. And though we may sleep right on the edge of our bed, we rarely roll off.

In fact, while the brain waves of a person in coma or under anesthesia are very slow and weak, our brain waves during sleep are often as perky as when we're fully awake!

This allows our sleeping brain to dream, organize and store memories, and even periodically scan the room for anything out of the ordinary. That's why we can be roused from sleep by the smell of smoke or a burglar's footsteps. And it's also why many babies find the stillness of our homes disquieting (it's oddly quiet compared with the constant rumble and jiggle they experienced in the womb).

MYTH 2: *During sleep, your body is at rest.*

FACT: Your muscles may be in repose during sleep, but your heart, lungs, and liver (and most other organs) work a twenty-four-hour shift. Even the brain is actively buzzing along during the REM (rapid eye movement) portion of sleep.

And on rare occasions, even our muscles switch on while we sleep! During night terrors, children quake and scream . . . despite being in deep slumber.

MYTH 3: *You're either awake . . . or asleep.*

FACT: Did you know that dolphins sleep with only half their brains at a time? (Sounds like a handy skill for new parents!) Well, the interesting thing is that we actually do something similar.

Researchers at the University of Wisconsin looked into the brain when exhaustion was approaching and found that some brain cells went to sleep while the rest stayed awake. In sleep-deprived rats, 10 percent of brain cells were fully in sleep mode even though the rodent was still *awake*.

This "microsleep" usually occurs when we stay awake too long. So the next time you find yourself squeezing diaper cream onto your toothbrush or tossing the laundry in the trash, just blame it on some weary brain cells deciding to call it a night while the rest of your brain is still finishing up the day's work.

MYTH 4: *The idea of "beauty sleep" is just a silly old wives' tale.*

FACT: If you want to look good, get more sleep! That's the conclusion of a recent European study. Casual observers were asked to pick out the best-looking people among a big stack of photos (some tired and some not) and they rated the well-rested men and women as being more attractive.

MYTH 5: *Our natural day/night cycle is twenty-four hours.*

FACT: It may sound a little like science fiction, but your brain doesn't want a twenty-four-hour day. It actually craves a twenty-five- to twenty-six-hour day!

In 1962, European researchers placed volunteers in an underground bunker totally isolated from the world. With no light cues from the outside or clocks to guide them, the volunteers quickly fell into daily day-night cycles lasting almost twenty-six hours.

What Is This Thing Called Sleep?

Nobody needs lessons in how to sleep . . . not even babies. (Though they may need some tutoring on *when* to sleep!)

For example, over the past fifty years, a very strange thing happened to our sleep: it shrank! The average adult nighttime sleep dropped from eight hours to about seven. In fact, the US Centers for Disease Control reported that 21 percent of adults sleep only six hours (and 8 percent sleep five hours or less!). Is that okay or is it hurting us? In truth, we don't really know. Even though we spend a third of our lives dozing, there are still many unanswered questions about this hazy state.

But, thanks to the growing field called sleep medicine, we're beginning to understand what sleep does *for* us—and what losing sleep does *to* us.

Birds Do It, Bees Do It: The Bounty of Sleep

Critters big and small—from flies to whales—curl up and sleep. Elephants doze for just four hours, lions snooze for twenty hours, and sheep sleep about eight hours a day! (Which makes you wonder what sheep count when they want to doze off!) Why is sleep so universally important?

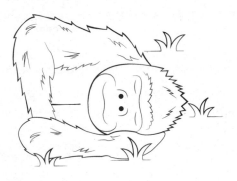

First, it replenishes us. Sleep restores the brain's alertness and the body's vigor.

Second, it boosts our health. Like a mysterious vitamin S, sleep strengthens our infection-fighting cells (that's why teens get sick when they pull an all-nighter); prevents depression; cuts heart disease in half; reduces obesity; and even stops cancer. (Ohio researchers found 50 percent more precancerous colon growths in people who routinely sleep less than six hours a night versus those sleeping more than seven.)

Finally, sleep allows the brain and body to tidy up and prepare for the next day. During sleep, our brains literally replay the events of the previous day; new experiences are compared with past recollections and memories are then revised and neatly filed away for later use.

This memory reorganization is at the heart of our ability to create new ideas. No wonder we say, "Let's sleep on it" and "Everything will make sense in the morning." It isn't the light of day that clears things up; it's the intense brain activity during sleep that lets trivial memories fade away and new solutions bubble up and take root in our conscious minds.

Sleep Cues: Easing into Sleep

Most animals are creatures of habit when it comes to where and how they sleep.

Gorillas love snoozing on nests of soft branches and leaves, bats like to doze in caves (hanging upside down by their toes), and most of us require a few very specific conditions to help us ease into slumber. Some need a soft bed or a special pillow or perhaps a heavy quilt. You might require total quiet, while your friend can only sleep with the TV on.

We call these helpful aids "sleep cues." And, as you will see in the coming chapters, some cues are magically wonderful for young children, while others lead you right down the road to disaster!

The High Cost of Lost Sleep

If you're the parent of a young child, you've already learned how quickly exhaustion builds when you're disturbed several times a night. Frequent waking keeps us swirling in light sleep and reduces the deep, restorative slumber that we need to prepare our bodies and minds for the challenges of the next day.

Chronic sleep deprivation makes:

Our mood drop. We get whiny, unhappy, and demanding.

Our coordination flop. We get klutzy, off-balance, and accident-prone.

Our thinking sink. We get forgetful and confused.

Our resilience crumble. We gain weight and suffer problems from pimples to cancer.

Exhaustion is such a stressful experience that the elite Navy SEALs are put through prolonged sleep deprivation to train them to endure torture!

We may be able to muddle through despite night after night of poor sleep, but it builds up a mounting "sleep debt" in the body and brain that eventually must be paid, either with some solid catch-up sleep . . . or with our health.

Mommy Brain: Your Head Takes an Unexpected Vacation

Have you ever seen the T-shirt that says OH MY GOD, I LEFT THE BABY ON THE BUS!?

Most new moms notice that their memory turns to mush right after giving birth (or even a few months before). Many women joke that part of their brain must have come out with the placenta, and nursing moms often complain of "milk brain." (Scientists have speculated that this memory holiday is Nature's blessed way of helping women forget the rigors of childbirth.)

And exhaustion makes this "brain fog" even worse!

Luckily, mommy brain resolves . . . eventually. A Dutch study found clunkier-than-normal thinking speed months after the birth. But Australian researchers found that years after childbirth, the brain works just as well as before pregnancy (except for difficulty remembering why their husband's jokes used to seem so hilarious).

Drunk—or Sleep Deprived?

A journalist friend said she got so tired when she became a mom that one day, when she went to pick up her infant at day care, she pulled into a parking space and then proceeded to continue driving her car right into the building!

The University of Pennsylvania's renowned sleep researcher David Dinges has probably robbed more people of sleep than anyone else in the world. In one experiment, he and his team allowed some volunteers to sleep only six hours a night while others got to snooze for eight hours.

During the day, the scientists tested all participants every two hours, measuring their ability to pay attention. The well-rested group stayed sharp, but the six-hour group became increasingly scattered and distractible. Two weeks into the study, the attention span of members of the six-hour group dropped to the level of people who were legally drunk!

And, also like being drunk, sleep deprivation causes poor judgment, slow reaction time, and impaired memory. When you're exhausted, you stagger, stutter, and slur your words. At its most extreme, sleep deprivation can even trigger hallucinations.

Alarmingly, the National Sleep Foundation's 2004 Sleep in America poll found that 48 percent of parents admitted to driving while drowsy, and 10 percent confessed to falling asleep at the wheel.

Beware the Caffeine Cure

You may recall from science class that the body's cells use a special fuel called ATP (adenosine triphosphate). As ATP is used in brain cells, it leaves behind a heap of plain adenosine. By the end of the day, so much adenosine builds up in each cell that it starts a chain reaction that creates "cobwebs" in our brains, forcing our minds to lose focus and our eyes to close.

That's where coffee can come to the rescue!

Caffeine blocks the brain from recognizing that adenosine levels are high, which stops that "I'm sleepy" message so you feel wide-awake. Caffeine also causes the release of adrenaline—providing a little jolt of nervous energy—and it boosts dopamine, one of the brain's natural "feel-good" chemicals.

Caffeine may seem like a tempting quick fix when you're short on sleep . . . but beware! It passes right into the breast milk and can cause your baby to become irritable and more awake.

Furthermore, caffeine lingers in the body for over twelve hours (a quarter of the caffeine from a noontime cup of coffee is still in your blood at midnight). This can keep you from being able to sink into deep sleep. And the fatigue from too little deep sleep may make you feel even *more* tired, irritable, and depressed and make you reach for even *more* caffeine the next day!

My suggestion? Limit your coffee to just a morning cup. If you're exhausted, try to take a nap, rather than mask your fatigue with caffeine (or with similar stimulants in tea, cola, energy drinks, supplements, or chocolate).

Fascinating Rhythm—Your Day/Night Circadian Cycle

As you can see, getting enough sleep is crucial. But that can be hard when you're struggling for hours to soothe a screaming baby or to persuade your wide-eyed toddler to go back into her room. In your frustration, you may be tempted to think your child is being willful and defiant, but there may be a biological factor undermining your child's sleep: the ticking of her inner clock.

The brain's inner clock orchestrates the beautiful flow of our bodies through waking and sleep. And knowing a bit of the science behind this process will give you key insights to help your child move smoothly through this daily dance. So let's take a closer look at the biology of this thing we call sleep.

All plants and animals dance to certain rhythms. Flowers open in the morning and fold their petals at night. Trees drop their leaves each fall and form buds that blossom in the spring, and bears hibernate every winter, emerging from sleep when the weather warms.

For humans (and most other land creatures), our most important biological rhythm is the twenty-four-hour cycle of day and night. Your body and brain closely mirror these repeating waves of light and dark, up and down, every day of your life. Scientists call these pulsations our *circadian rhythm* (from Latin for "about one day").

We tend to take the circadian rhythm for granted. But imagine what life would be like without this internal clock keeping us in sync with the sun. One day, we'd fall asleep in the inky black of ten o'clock at night. The next day we might doze off during the bright light at one o'clock in the afternoon. And we might sleep for five hours on Monday and fifteen on Tuesday. It would be chaos!

Fortunately, our circadian rhythm helps us perfectly follow the sun's cycles. Like a silently ticking internal, biological clock, this rhythm wakes us with the light of the morning and delivers us into sleep every night. (We may change what time we "hit the hay" and "rise and shine," but the circadian rhythm still demands that our sleep plus wake hours always total twenty-four hours each day.)

Let There Not Be Light

Our circadian clock controls our day/night cycle through the release of a powerful sleep-inducing signal, the hormone melatonin.

Here's how it works. When light reaches the retina (the back surface of the eye), it sends a signal directly to a pair of pinhead-sized structures located back behind the eyes. These structures, the epicenter of our ancient biological clock, are called the suprachiasmatic nuclei, or SCN.

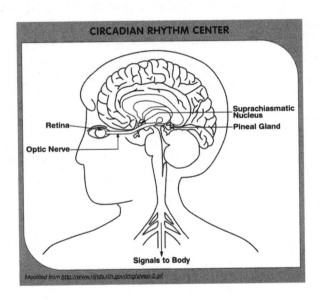

The SCN then shoots an "it's daytime" signal to a structure deep in the brain, the tiny pineal gland, which dutifully shuts off the production of melatonin. This continues for as long as the sun is shining. Then as darkness comes, the SCN stops getting the light signal and shoots an "it's nighttime" message to the pineal gland to prompt it to release melatonin, which—like a natural sleeping potion—quickly induces drowsiness.

By now, you've noticed that the major player in this cycle is light.

Even a little bit of light (such as a streetlamp outside your bedroom window) can pass right through your closed eyelids, sending your SCN a wake-up call and shutting off melatonin, which makes getting into sleep a challenge.

This is why people in Alaska (with twenty-two-hour days in summer and twenty-two-hour nights in winter) have trouble getting into good sleep schedules. And it's also why bright lights in your home after dark (lamps, TV, or computer screens . . . even your cell phone) can wreak havoc on your sleep.

And once we are asleep, the circadian rhythm gives way to another cycle that then organizes and orchestrates our slumber, the roller-coaster fluctuations between REM and non-REM sleep.

The Ancient Greeks on Sleep

Hypnos was the god of sleep in Greek mythology. He was the son of Nyx (Night) and he lived in the land of eternal darkness, far beyond the gates of the rising sun. Each night, he flew through the dark sky spreading the gift of sleep (even to other gods).

According to the ancient Greeks Hypnos's brothers included Momus (Blame), Nemesis (Envy), Geras (Old Age), and Thanatos (Peaceful Death).

And, as you might have guessed, Hypnos was also father to Morpheus, god of dreams. (Morpheus's mom was Pasithea, the goddess of hallucination.)

Morpheus could take any form in people's dreams. His regal domain was located right next to the River of Forgetfulness, and was protected by two terrible monsters that repelled intruders by turning into the visitor's deepest fears. (Modern medicine

A Tale of Two Sleeps—REM and NREM

You'll have a better understanding of your child's sleep if you understand how your own sleep works. So here's a closer look at the two special types of sleep that take turns controlling our brains while we sleep.

For centuries, people thought of sleep as a long, formless marshmallow of tranquility. But about sixty years ago, we accidentally discovered that it is much more interesting than that.

In 1953, researchers watching infants sleep noticed that every so often the babies' eyes skittered under their closed lids. (Watch your baby sleeping—so much fun! You'll notice these funny movements come and go, along with little smiles and faster breathing.)

This observation was our first proof that sleep is not one continuous clump from dark to dawn. It is actually made up of repeating cycles of two very different types of sleep: REM, when our eyes dance as if we're watching a video on the inside of the eyelids; and non-REM (NREM), when our eyes are totally still.

When we doze off, the brain usually goes right into NREM sleep, for some well-deserved rest. About every ninety minutes our sleep completes one cycle, passing from light sleep to deep sleep and then returning to light sleep, or even a brief waking. This is usually followed by a five- to twenty-minute slab of REM sleep to complete one cycle. Our brains string together four to five of these to create one night's sleep.

This pattern can be seen in the figure on page 19. This diagram is called a hypnogram. As you can see, there are repeating appearances of deep and light NREM sleep. The first cycles have little REM, but toward morning, REM increases and deep sleep lessens. Just before waking, sleep is usually pure REM alternating with light sleep (that's why our dreams are often the most vivid when we're accidentally awakened a little early).

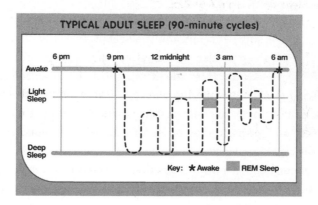

NREM—a Closer Look at the Restful Type of Sleep

Each night adults spend about 85 percent of our slumber in NREM sleep. As mentioned, this is the period of sleep that restores and refreshes the body and brain. NREM sleep is divided into three stages—light, medium, and deep. Here's what happens in each one.

Stage 1—Drowsiness or "Just Nodding Off"

Ahh, your mind is beginning to relax. You miss some of the TV show you're watching . . . until you feel a little jerk of your head and return to wakefulness. If asked, you'd probably say you were just daydreaming.

Stage 1 usually lasts ten to twenty minutes.

Stage 2— Light Sleep

You're sleeping, but you wake easily if someone calls your name or jostles you. And when you wake, you definitely know you were just asleep.

Stage 2 usually lasts twenty to thirty minutes.

Stage 3—Deep, or "Slow Wave," Sleep

Stage 3 NREM is the most refreshing: the sleep sweet spot! You're sleeping like a log. Breathing is slow and regular, and your face and body are relaxed but not floppy. Lift your child's arm when she's in stage 3 and it will slowly drift back to the mattress. (In deep NREM, some kids and adults sweat profusely on their heads.)

Stage 3 sleep is also called "slow wave" sleep because your brain waves switch from the jittering little bounces seen during waking to slow, undulating waves. These waves wash over the brain 1000 times a night, erasing memories from the day just passed and preparing the brain for a new day of learning. In this deepest of sleep, you're tough to rouse—and when you do wake up, you may need a minute or two to figure out where you are.

Stage 3 is very deep, which is why it's also the sleep stage when exhausted parents accidentally overlay and suffocate their bed-sharing baby. However, it is definitely not coma. You can still wake for important signals, like a smoke alarm or your baby's cry.

When you're rising back up from deep sleep, a strange thing can happen. Your muscle control may start to back up while the rest of your brain is still deep in twinkle land. This is exactly when bizarre events like sleep talking or night terrors suddenly appear. In essence, part of the brain is awake while the rest is still in deep slumber.

Stage 3 usually lasts twenty to forty minutes.

Note: If your baby's squeaks and squawks wake you up every couple of hours, you may get seven hours of sleep yet feel as pooped as if you barely got four. That's because your brain is getting stuck in light sleep. It just never gets the chance to make the slow descent into deep, stage 3 NREM.

As stage 3 ends, your brain slowly bubbles back up to light, drowsy stage 1 sleep. That's when you're sensitive to anything amiss in your environment, like a passing motorcycle. But once you decide that all is copacetic, you usually glide back into sleep—not even remembering that you were awake.

Waking Up at 2 A.M.
Is a Smart Idea? Yup!

Videotapes reveal that we have many "miniwakings" throughout the night. We shift position, rearrange our pillow or grab our teddy, and then dive back into sleep. That's a good way to prevent bed sores or stiff joints.

These brief awakenings also benefit us as part of a . . . natural alarm system.

Think about this from your ancient ancestors' point of view. They lived in caves and small encampments, which made them vulnerable to nighttime intruders. Sleeping with "one eye open" would have been helpful, but obviously that can't be done. So the next best survival aid was to have each member of the family take a turn popping into near arousal every ninety minutes at the end of a sleep cycle.

Since each person would fall asleep at a slightly different time, large families were bound to have at least one member in light sleep—thus more vigilant to intruders—at any given time of the night. "Taking turns" in light sleep may have made the difference between life and death.

REM Sleep—a Closer Look at Dream/Memory Sleep

We spend about 15 percent of each night in REM sleep. REM is the land of dreams and memories. During REM sleep breathing is irregular, the face is visited by tiny smiles and grimaces, and the muscles are loose and floppy. Amazingly, the brain's electrical activity is almost as active as when we're fully awake! Yet, despite all this brain activity, in REM the brain ignores many of its jobs (hearing, vision, and sending movement commands to the muscles below the neck).

These changes allow us to focus on what we see and hear *in our dreams*. And, even though we may be dreaming we can fly, we're kept safe because the brain's commands to the muscles—to open the window and start flapping—are blocked.

When REM sleep is over and dreaming stops, the brain enters non-REM sleep and the blockade between the brain and body ends. (That's why sleepwalking can occur in NREM, but couldn't possibly occur during a dream about walking in REM sleep.)

Besides being a Mardi Gras of dream, REM is also when the brain scans the events of the day, compares them with past memories, and re-forms and re-files them as fresh new memories.

REM is extraordinary—it creates dreams that evaporate seconds after we wake, yet preserves and protects our memories to last a lifetime!

REM lasts five to ten minutes during sleep's first REM period and can last up to thirty minutes during the final hours of sleep.

Kid Sleep: What's Different and What's Not

So why is this science lesson relevant to *your* life? Well, if you compare everything we just learned with how babies and toddlers sleep, you'll see why going to bed (and staying there) is often more of a challenge for them.

Of course, kids and adults have lots of sleep similarities. For instance, we both:

- Yawn when we're tired.

- Have accidents when we're exhausted.

- Prefer sleeping at night (okay . . . this one may take a little time to happen).

- Love our own special sleep cues (from swaddling, white noise, and teddy bears to favorite pillows and flannel sheets).

But there are also key differences between adult and childhood sleep.

For one thing, kids sleep a lot more. Babies rack up fourteen to eighteen hours of slumber, although it's sprinkled in little bits throughout the night and day. Somewhere between the second and sixth month, day sleep coalesces into one- to two-hour naps, and night sleep forms blocks of six to ten hours.

During the toddler years, total daily sleep gradually drifts down to eleven or twelve hours (with naps of one to two hours) for a two-year-old. And then drops to ten or eleven hours (with no naps) for a five-year-old.

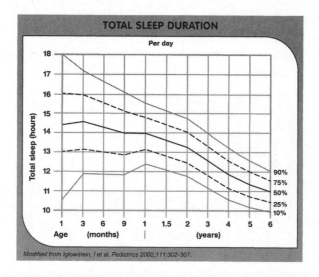

Kids also doze off earlier than grown-ups. Babies fall asleep between 9 and 10 P.M., and from six months to six years of age, infants sack out between 8 and 9 P.M. (The earliest bedtimes belong to eighteen- to twenty-three-month-olds, who often get tucked in around 8 P.M.)

Another pivotal difference is that a single adult sleep cycle lasts ninety minutes, while, as you can see in the next graph, young children zip through a cycle (from light to deep sleep and back to light, with a bit of REM tacked on) in just sixty minutes.

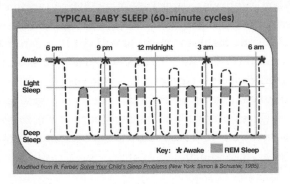

These shorter cycles will have a huge impact on your life. Why? Because speedier cycles mean that your child will return to very light—easily disturbed—sleep every hour. No wonder little kids are so easily disturbed by a little hunger or teething.

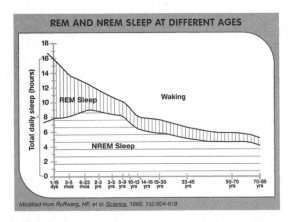

Finally, as shown in the graph above, your mix of NREM and REM is very different from your child's. We spend about 85 percent of the night in restorative NREM, babies spend just 50 percent in NREM (this is when kids can even snooze through roaring basketball games). On the other hand, babies spend a massive 40–50 percent of their sleep in dream/memory-boosting REM (versus about 15 percent in adults).

In other words, infants have five times more REM sleep than adults (8 hours versus 1.5). This gives them enough time to sift through all the day's chaotic happenings to figure out which new memories to file away and which ones to forget.

Adults probably need much less REM because our lives are pretty routine. Most of the things we encounter each day—like finding which grocery store aisle has dog food—are either not new to us or just too trivial to remember. But for babies, everything is new and fascinating. ("Wow . . . a hat! I've never seen one of those before. Ha-ha! It looks like Mommy's head just got superhuge!")

In fact, our little buddies' brains quickly fill to the brim with all the cool things they want to remember (like the bell on the cat's neck, the first swing ride, the ceiling fan, and the smell of fresh cookies). No wonder infants need to nap every few hours. Unlike adults, who first enter restorative sleep before we move on to REM, young kids dive immediately into REM to process their inbox of memories.

But how much of all this REM sleep is actually filled with infant dreams?

Do Little Kids Dream?

Little kids have tons of REM. So it's logical to assume that they must have all sorts of exciting kiddy-type dreams, like colossal smiling faces, giant-tongued dogs licking their toes, and breasts the size of blimps gushing sweet, warm milk.

Of course, babies can't speak, so it's impossible to know their dreams (or even if they're dreaming at all). But what about older kids?

Psychologist David Foulkes has worked with children (from tots to teens) to bring the secrets of their dreams to the light of day. In his lab, he allows children to fall asleep and then wakes them three times a night—sometimes in REM and sometimes in NREM—and asks them to describe what they're thinking.

Foulkes's findings are surprising . . . in how unsurprising they are.

Basically, immature kids have immature dreams. For children under five, dreams are usually just static visions of an animal or bland images of people eating and doing other mundane activities.

Interestingly preschoolers often think their dreams are magically placed in their heads by someone else, or by God.

Most of us remember bits and pieces of our waking activities starting from around three or four years of age, but our earliest dream memories usually start at six or seven years (even though we have tons of REM sleep before that). When roused during REM sleep, 25 percent of kids under nine years of age have no recollection of dreaming.

Lastly, kids' dreams are happier than adults'! In contrast to grown-up dreams (which usually contain aggression and misfortune), Foulkes found that children's dreams are embroidered with happy emotions.

Why Do We Yawn When We See Babies Yawn?

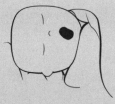

Dogs yawn . . . and cats and monkeys . . . and even three-month-old fetuses (but not chickens).

An average yawn lasts four to six seconds. We yawn more when we're tired or bored. And trying to make it stop usually just makes another yawn pop right out. But surprisingly, we have no idea why we yawn. It's a big medical mystery.

We also have no idea why yawns are so contagious. At around four years of age, we develop an irresistible urge to join in when we see others yawning. Children with autism, however, are an exception. The more severe a child's autism, the less likely he or she is to catch another person's yawn.

Back to the Real World—and an Epidemic of Sleeplessness

I hope this quick look at the world of sleep was informative. Understanding sleep cycles and the biology of slumber will be helpful if your child develops sleep problems. And sadly, there's a good chance that he or she will.

As these charts from the National Sleep Foundation's 2004 Sleep in America Survey show, 60 to 80 percent of parents report that their young child has a sleep problem at least a few days a week. The biggest struggles are around resistance going to bed and trouble falling asleep.

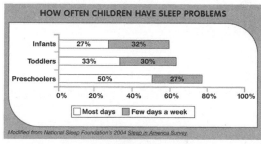

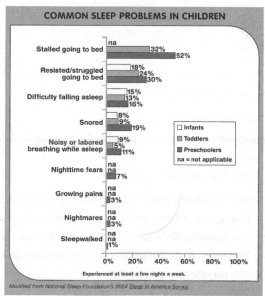

If that sounds like your situation and you're tired, edgy, and your confidence is shaken, good sleep may be closer than you think! And it shouldn't require "tough love" or hours of crying (your baby's or yours).

In the next chapters, I'll discuss sleep problems at three different ages: the first three months of life, later infancy, and the toddler/preschool years. You'll learn whether your little one has a sleep problem . . . and if the answer is yes, I hope to convince you that the cure is much easier than you thought.

## PART I

Sweet Sleep for Little Babies: Birth to Three Months

Chapter 2 is all about setting the stage for safe and happy sleep. You'll learn how your baby's amazing brain changes during the first three months and how these changes affect his sleep. Then I'll shed light on the top ten myths about baby sleep and discuss how much sleep you can realistically expect in those first months. I'll tackle one of the biggest controversies in parenting—should you bed-share? And finally, I'll list the top ways to reduce your baby's risk of SIDS or suffocation.

Chapter 3 shares a handful of *Happiest Baby* way tips to help you guide your little one from screaming to calm . . . usually in just minutes (or less). You'll learn how to enhance sleep by using the *5 S*'s to trigger your baby's *calming reflex*, and you'll discover why waking your sleeping baby isn't crazy—it's smart. I'll give tips on scheduling your baby's day, and finally I'll review how to boost the sleep of preemies and multiples.

Chapter 4 gives feeding advice to help your sweetie sleep a little longer. I'll provide tips for preventing illnesses that can disrupt sleep and for helping your little one cope if she does get a cough or sniffle. Finally, you'll learn the key signs of postpartum depression (and the steps you can take to help prevent it).

Chapter 5 gives the answers to sleep questions that many new moms and dads worry about.

## CHAPTER TWO

The Early Days: Setting the Stage for Safe and Happy Sleep

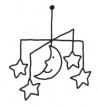

KEY POINTS:

★ Your baby's personality affects how she acts when she's awake . . . and it also affects how well she sleeps.

★ Good sleep starts with good *state control*—your baby's ability to calm her own crying and stay asleep despite lights and noises.

★ New babies have an amazing ability to learn, which allows us to quickly teach them to sleep better and longer.

- ★ Debunking the top myths about baby sleep will help you avoid mistakes as you strive to promote better slumber.

- ★ Your top job is to keep your little one safe—which includes taking steps to prevent SIDS and suffocation. And that's why bed-sharing is a risk you're smart to avoid in the early months.

A journey of a thousand miles begins with a single (baby) step.

—ADAPTED FROM LAO-TZU

Kid Stuff: What's Going On in Your Baby's Mind?

Why does your friend's baby fall asleep fast while yours screams through the night? Are you doing something wrong? Is your friend a gifted parent? Are you a total flop?

No!

In this chapter, you'll learn that each baby is unique. Some lucky parents have newborns who sleep great no matter what. But, if yours is a bit tougher, welcome to the club! Millions of other sleep-deprived moms and dads just like you are pacing the floor at this very moment, all around the world.

However, that doesn't mean you're doomed to months of exhaustion. In this section, you'll discover some *Happiest Baby* ways to help your little lamb sleep like . . . a little lamb. If you're brand-new to this approach, I think you'll be surprised at how easy it is to switch off most of your baby's screaming and switch on her happy sleep. And, if you're already familiar with the *Happiest Baby*, I'll share some new wrinkles to transform these tips into a no-tears way to teach babies to sleep better, starting as early as one week of age. (Really!)

But first, good sleep begins with understanding what's going on in your baby's mind. And that starts with knowing about a few key traits that have a big effect on sleeping: temperament, state control, and learning.

Temperament—The Sea Your Child Sails On

I recently ran into Tia, mother of three, in a coffee shop. With her was Sophia, her beautiful and talented eighteen-year-old. With a big smile, Tia reminded me that when Sophia was ten days old, as I held her on my lap I mentioned that it took extra bouncing and vigor to settle her down. Tia said she remembered me remarking, "Wow! I wouldn't be surprised if this girl loves sports and roller coasters when she grows up." Then she laughed and proclaimed that both predictions were right on target.

Much of a person's demeanor is a genetic "hand-me-down" from his mom and dad. Like blue eyes and curly hair, a baby's temperament is a roll of the "personality dice" with some (or a lot) of the child's charisma or caution coming directly from her parents. That's why shy parents often have shy children, and passionate parents often have little chili peppers.

In all honesty, predicting a baby's temperament—as I did with Sophia—is a very imprecise science. But after thirty years of taking care of babies, I've observed that some personality—or temperament—qualities can often be seen in the first weeks.

A smooth sea (calm temperament) helps babies breeze through infancy. These infants are sunny and happy and easy to soothe. Mellow and mild, they squeak rather than shriek, as if patiently saying, "Please, Mummy, I'm a bit hungry."

But a choppy sea (a cautious or spirited temperament) makes for some rough times (colic, frequent waking, refusing a pacifier) until a child is mature enough to manage her hypersensitivity and tidal waves of passion.

Cautious babies cry when you laugh too loud and give Grandma the cold shoulder if her perfume is too strong. These wide-eyed babes are as transparent and pure as crystal. But like crystal, they're supersensitive and fragile. Once mature, they're a wonder to be around, creative and highly perceptive. But as infants they're slow to warm, easily overloaded, and their own startle can unleash rivers of sobbing.

Spirited babies, on the other hand, are superintense and easily unbalanced. They rapidly develop glass-shattering screams and tornadolike moods. And when the sparks of everyday frustration touch the dynamite of their explosive temperament, KAPOW! As infants, these kids struggle to keep their balance. But as they get a bit older, they develop waves of wonderful giggling, intense curiosity, and boundless enthusiasm.

Just as it affects your baby's behavior in the daytime, temperament can also create nighttime problems.

Sensitive babies often wake because they're bothered by outside disturbances (lights, sounds, etc.) or internal discomforts (teething, hunger, etc.). And they can be very picky about the white noise you choose to help them sleep, ignoring it if it's too mellow (like ocean waves) or getting upset by noise that's too sharp and hissy (like fans and air filters).

Spirited kids fall apart when they're overtired. A spirited babe might yell for milk . . . and then keep on crying even after the breast or bottle is in his mouth!

Understanding your tot's temperament is key to figuring out why she acts the way she does—and why she struggles with sleep. ("Oh, she always has trouble sleeping at Grandma's. The room is too bright." "She's so intense, once she starts crying she'll scream for an hour . . . and then vomit!") But don't worry: you will soon learn some very specific steps to help even the shyest or most spirited baby become a great sleeper.

State Control—Tuning the World In . . . or Shutting It Out

"My one-month-old is so much fun to watch," said Britta. "Bobby's little lip quivers when he's upset. He's clearly trying to hold back the flood of tears, and he can go a long time making a silly meow-type cry before he loses the battle and goes ballistic."

If temperament is the sea your little one sails on, state control tells you how steady (or jumpy) his boat is.

Can your little one stay asleep despite mild hunger and jarring noise? Does his fussing always lead to an escalating upset, or can he usually settle down from crying . . . all by himself?

These are signs of your baby's state control.

In this context, the word *state* refers to a baby's level of alertness (not to whether he lives in Maine or Alabama). Your baby spends the day moving between six states of gradually increasing awakeness and vigor: deep sleep, light sleep, drowsiness, quiet alertness, fussiness, and screaming. Smoothly controlling these (not jumping from one to another) is one of his brain's first big jobs.

(Notice that right in the middle of the six is quiet alertness. In this magical state your baby's eyes will be bright and open and his face will be relaxed as he thoughtfully studies the sights all around him.)

Good "self-calmers" gracefully shift between sleep and alertness and are surprisingly good at gearing down from fussing to quiet . . . all on their own. And when the world gets too wild, they have an uncanny ability to protect themselves from getting overwhelmed: they stare into space, look away (as we do at a scary movie), or simply retreat into sleep.

How State Control Helps Your Baby Stay Asleep

This little experiment shows how your baby's state control is the secret to his amazing "sleep anywhere, anytime" ability.

Get a flashlight and tiptoe in while your baby is sleeping. Shine the light right on his closed eyes for one or two seconds. He'll probably tighten his closed eyes, stir a bit, and breathe faster (or maybe even startle).

Wait a few seconds to allow him to settle back into sleep. Then shine the light on his eyes again. He'll probably react as before, or a little less.

Repeat this a few times and you'll see something very interesting: after three or four flashes, his responses will lessen greatly, and after three or four more, he may have no reaction at all. That's a sign that his state control is protecting him by stopping his brain from paying attention to the light!

Clearly, your baby's brain doesn't "shut off" during sleep. It's still working, doing its best to ignore disturbances. Many of the tricks you'll learn in this book are designed to boost state control and help your baby tune out distractions and stay settled in peaceful sleep.

On the other hand, some babies (including many preemies or those born to drug users) have unsteady, immature state control. They startle a lot, and they have trouble screening out even the normal commotions. Their shrieks are often their way of begging for help: "Please . . . pick me up . . . the world is too big!"

For decades, smart nurses have known that these babies desperately need swaddling, shushing, and rocking. Infants with poor state control depend on us to keep their calming reflex turned on until they get old enough to settle their crying jags on their own.

State control also explains one more mystery: why many babies cry more around dinnertime (the so-called witching hour). Late in the day, babies with shaky state control just can't "keep it together" after a full day of exciting activity (and far too little soothing holding, rocking, and sucking). Their ability to keep their boat steady gets overwhelmed, and they just disintegrate into tearful, flailing little furies.

Don't worry if your baby has poor state control; he'll grow out of it. But it does mean that as a parent you might need to work harder to calm him and get him to sleep. Fortunately, a few tricks will help even the most jittery baby become a sound sleeper. (In the next two chapters, you'll find out exactly how.)

Learning—Your Baby's Amazing Ability to Remember

You've probably noticed times when your baby's chin trembled, or her eyes crossed. Newborns pretty much have the coordination of drunken sailors. Although only *some* babies have immature state control, they *all* have immature muscle control. Not all animals have such puny offspring. Baby horses, for example, can run on the first day of life. So why are our babies so babyish?

It's simple: humans have a narrow pelvis. That helps us walk and run well (much easier with legs that are right next to each other, not widely separated). But it makes delivering a baby's big head a very tough squeeze. We all want smart babies, but we don't want their brains getting big until after they're born!

Imagine you're taking a long trip but can bring only one suitcase. That's your baby's dilemma. Her small head has to fit through the birth canal, so she can only pack it with the things she'll absolutely need to survive in the outside world . . . the bare essentials.

Over the millennia, Nature has picked four totally indispensable abilities to take up the majority of space in our babies' orange-sized brains:

- **Life support controls—heart rate, blood pressure, breathing, and so on**

- **State control—turning attention on (to interact with the world) and off (to recover and sleep)**

- **Reflexes—built-in "software" that helps babies do complex things like sneeze, suck, swallow, and cry**

- **Muscle/sense control (a little bit)—the ability to touch, taste, look at, and interact with the world**

For the first few weeks, these abilities pretty much restrict your baby's daily activities to eating, looking, sleeping, peeing, and pooping.

Yet, as limited as your baby's brain is, it has one more truly surprising talent . . . the ability to learn!

Our little ones begin to recognize the voices and music they hear in the womb. And after birth, babies quickly learn to distinguish the scent of their mom's milk from another mom's. They also learn to coo and squirm the moment they see Dad's smiling face . . . even before his tickling finger starts poking them.

As I mentioned earlier, this learning—sifting through and filing away each day's huge siloful of new experiences—is probably why babies have five times more REM sleep than we do.

Since babies are such great learners, you'd think they ought to be able to learn to sleep better. In fact, they can! Teaching your baby good sleep cues is key to helping her snooze better (and it's equally important not to accidentally teach unwanted cues, like being rocked all night long).

Generations of sleep experts have claimed that babies can't be trained to sleep until they reach three to four months of age. Well, that's simply not true . . . it's a myth! And it's just one of the many myths that I want to dispel.

Don't Believe It! Common Myths About Baby Sleep

You'd think since we've been around babies—forever!—we'd pretty much know everything about them. But beware: the more books you read and grandmas you talk with, the more sleep misunderstandings and misperceptions you'll encounter.

Here's one big myth: "New parents are supposed to raise their baby all on their own."

Nonsense! Throughout history, new parents have relied on tons of help. Family and friends in most cultures around the world have always "mothered the mother"—until recently, when a ridiculous myth was launched: "You're a *wuss* if you need a nanny, and incompetent if you need your family's help."

Fact: Raising kids *does* take a village! So right now is the perfect time to pull in favors. Of course, you should be prepared to return those favors when your friends and family need help from you.

And speaking of myths, here are the top ten mistaken baby sleep ideas you're likely to hear from the moms you meet in the park.

MYTH 1: *Babies are naturally good sleepers.*

FACT: Don't let the phrase "sleeping like a baby" fool you. Babies sleep a lot, but it's broken into bits and pieces throughout the day. And sometimes, just like adults, babies *party too hard.* They can get so excited by your home's daily commotion that they stay up too long . . . which makes them wired and miserable and makes it even harder for them to *leave the party* and give in to sleep.

MYTH 2: *Never wake a sleeping baby.*

FACT: Sometimes it's essential to wake your baby up! For example, if she poops in her sleep, you need to wake her to change her diaper in order to protect her skin. And waking her up for an 11 P.M. *dream feed* (an extra couple of ounces) may be to the key step in improving her sleep.

Moreover, intentionally waking your baby is an essential step in teaching her the skill of self-soothing (falling back to sleep on his or her own after being jolted awake by a ringing phone or passing truck).

And don't worry. You'll be able to help her slide back into sleep in no time even before she learns self-soothing once you master the skill of turning on her *calming reflex.*

MYTH 3: *Sleeping babies need us to tiptoe around.*

FACT: *You* may like sleeping in peace and quiet, but for your baby, it's really weird! That's because in the womb, she was surrounded by a

24/7 symphony of sensations—holding, soft touch, loud whooshing, and lots of jiggling.

So sleeping in stillness is actually a form of sensory deprivation to a baby . . . like locking us in a dark closet!

Of course, chaotic disturbances—like clanging pots—will disturb your baby's sleep. But rhythmic jiggly motion and the right white noise sound (rumbling and low pitched) will be two of your top tools for boosting her naps and nights.

MYTH 4: *Rocking your baby to sleep every night will make her dependent on it.*

FACT: Well, this one is a little trickier.

It's true that rocking and nursing your baby to sleep every night will delay her learning how to get to sleep on her own. However, rocking and nursing your baby to sleep is absolutely delicious and will probably become one of your most treasured memories of these early days. (And babies are held and rocked nonstop in the womb—so your little friend is already "hooked" on these sleep cues from before Day 1.)

Fortunately, it's supereasy to enjoy as much holding, nursing, and rocking as you want, without causing sleep problems. All you need to do is add other soothing sensations to your bedtime mix (like white noise and swaddling) and use the quick "wake and sleep" technique (which I'll teach you soon) to turn your baby into an excellent self-soother.

MYTH 5: *Colic is crying caused by mysterious stomach pains.*

FACT: For thousands of years, colic (sudden screaming fits that total three or more hours a day) has been a medical mystery. This crying starts at two to three weeks, hits a peak at six to eight weeks, and then gradually disappears by about three months. But, the fact that most screaming babies can be quickly calmed with the 5 S's shows this crying isn't caused by pain.

Doctors and grandmas have always assumed colicky babies were upset from stomach pain—overfeeding, indigestion, or acid reflux pain. Although some do grunt and fuss right after a feeding—and 5 to 10 percent get better with a change in formula or their mom's diet—it is now clear that this daily wailing is *not* caused by stomach pain.

How can I be so sure? For a bunch of reasons:

- **Ninety percent of fussy babies show no benefit from dietary change.**

- **The crying often improves with vacuum cleaner sounds or bumpy car rides. Yet loud noise or cruising the interstate does nothing to relieve severe pain. (It certainly wouldn't help *our* stomachs!)**

- **Most colicky babies calm in minutes—or less—when their parents correctly imitate the womb sensations. (I'll talk much more about how to do this by using the *5 S*'s to turn on the *calming reflex* in the next chapter.)**

MYTH 6: *Letting your baby cry to "blow off steam" is healthy.*

FACT: Psychologist Lee Salk said it best: "Crying is good for the lungs the way bleeding is good for the veins!" I totally agree. Just because your baby is capable of screaming doesn't mean it's beneficial for him to go on and on.

The idea that wee ones need to scream to exercise their lungs or to "blow off steam" to unwind from the day's chaos makes no sense, biologically or emotionally. First, crying is not a lung exercise (the lungs of calm babies are just as strong as those of colicky babies). Second, letting your baby "cry it out" is as crazy as ignoring your screeching car alarm while you wait for the battery to go dead.

Young infants only cry for one reason: they need help! The solution is to figure out how to meet their need.

MYTH 7: *Some babies hate swaddling.*

FACT: It sure looks like some babies hate swaddling! They fight and strain as soon as they're enveloped. But remember, in the womb, babies are perfectly content . . . yet they have *no freedom to move.*

As I'll describe in the section on swaddling, your baby may struggle when her arms are snugly straightened into the wrap. But then, when you add the other special steps that switch on her amazing *calming reflex* she'll tend to soothe quickly, stay calm longer, and sleep better.

MYTH 8: *We should teach babies to sleep in their own room.*

FACT: We all want our babies to grow up to be independent. But that's a goal that will take a long time to achieve—as any parent of a fifteen-year-old will tell you!

In truth, having your baby sleep in another room during the first months is inconvenient—and may even be a danger. It's inconvenient because you have to leave your warm bed and stumble down a cold hall every time your hungry baby cries. And it's a danger because sleeping in the same room can reduce a baby's risk of sudden infant death syndrome (also known as SIDS).

MYTH 9: *Your baby needs to adapt to the family, not the family to your baby.*

FACT: This one is sooooo wrong.

As your little girl gets closer to her first birthday, teaching limits will definitely become a major parenting objective, but for now your main goals are to build her confidence and trust in you. Feeling secure is a *much* earlier priority for little kids than feeling independent.

Remember, in the womb, you rocked and carried (and fed) your baby every single second. So during the first months, even if you hold her twelve hours a day, that's an immediate 50 percent cutback—from her point of view.

I want every child to learn good table manners, but it's crazy trying to teach them to a six-month-old. As the Bible says, "To everything there is a season." And now is the season for cuddling your sweet, kissable baby and making her feel protected and loved. There will be plenty of time for training and discipline in the months ahead.

MYTH 10: *It takes months for babies to learn to sleep well at night.*

FACT: Many parenting books perpetuate this myth. They state that a baby's brain is too immature to learn to sleep six hours before the age of three to four months. But I disagree.

As you now know, babies are learning even in the womb! And with a few simple tips, you can help your little one sleep hours longer in just weeks, not months.

And now that you know the myths, let's get on to the facts about babies and sleep.

Setting the Stage

Most likely, you have a houseful of baby gifts—from blankets and bottles to toys and teddy bears. But one of the best gifts you can give your baby is a perfect sleep environment.

Once you understand your little mouse's sleep needs and how to create a bedtime setting that's snug and safe, you'll be able to give her a great start on a lifetime of great sleep. Ready for some fun? Let's go!

What's Normal Sleep for a Newborn?

Babies may be too short to compete in the Olympics, but they definitely hold the world's record for championship sleeping. With an average of sixteen hours a day (and, rarely, up to twenty!), babies rack up more snoozing than at any other time in life.

Yet this can be a fooler! You'd think that sixteen hours of baby sleep would leave you tons of free time every day. But newborn sleep is shredded into confetti-like bits sprinkled throughout the light and night. It's like winning the lottery—but getting paid in pennies.

And if your child only needs twelve or thirteen hours of sleep per day, it's even crazier. Between feeding, bathing, diaper changes, and calming crying—God help you—it can feel like you never get a break.

And many parents are surprised by their *newborn's* sleep pattern. During the first day of life, most babies are alert for about an hour and then they can fall into deep sleep for twelve to eighteen hours. (Like most of us, they're exhausted by the whole ordeal.)

Of course, you should cuddle your baby during this period (skin-to-skin is great) and offer feedings—but even if she suckles, the breasts contain very little milk on the first day. Don't worry, however! Your early milk (colostrum) is rich in protein, antibodies, and nutrients to get your baby off to a great start. Additionally, like a little camel, your baby is born with an extra pound of food and water in her body.

Over the next day or two, your baby will become increasingly awake and hungry and begin the classic pattern—awake for one to two hours, then sleeping for two to four—that will dominate her life for the first month.

Naturally, since your baby wakes frequently in the first two months, so will you. And that's a problem because when you wake frequently, you end up getting twice as much light sleep and just half as much deep, restorative sleep. That's why you may still feel exhausted when you wake up in the morning. (This can be especially tough if you slept poorly the last months of pregnancy or are recovering from a C-section.)

Luckily, even in the first weeks, the *Happiest Baby* tips will help you get an hour or two of extra rest. So if you're feeling like a walking zombie, hang in there . . . relief is on the way!

You can also boost your mood (and save your sanity) by taking good care of yourself: get a little sun and exercise each morning; avoid junk food; and nap thirty to sixty minutes a day. (Many moms say it's easiest to sleep between 3 and 5 P.M., and hardest between 5 and 7 P.M.)

Every baby is different. Here are some typical sleep/wake/feed schedules that you might experience with your three-week-old and two-month-old. (You can find a list of sample sleep schedules for children from birth to four years in the back of this book.)

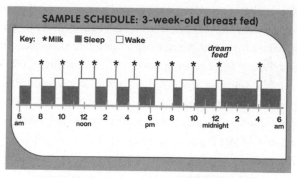

Daytime starts: 7 am
Night sleep starts: 10 pm
# of feeds/24 hrs: 9-12
# of naps/24 hrs: 3-6

Daytime sleep: 5-8 hrs
Longest night sleep: 3-5 hrs
Total night sleep: 7-8 hrs
Total sleep/24 hrs: 12-16 hrs

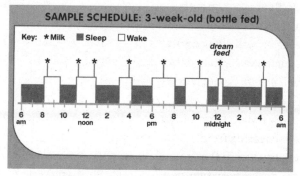

Daytime starts: 7 am
Night sleep starts: 10 pm
# of feeds/24 hrs: 7-10
# of naps/24 hrs: 4-6

Daytime sleep: 5-8 hrs
Longest night sleep: 4-5 hrs
Total night sleep: 7-8 hrs
Total sleep/24 hrs: 12-16 hrs

Location, Location, Location: Where Should Your Baby Sleep?

One of the first questions you have to answer after you give birth is, *Where will my baby sleep?*

A bassinet? Crib? Cosleeper? Your bed?

It's a decision that deserves some serious thought because it will affect your sleep, your baby's sleep, and your baby's safety.

Hands down, having your newborn baby sleep in your room is the way to go! It's cozier and *much* more convenient. It lets you hear when your baby spits up, has breathing troubles, or is uncomfortable in any way. And, as a total bonus, your being close by reduces her SIDS risk. So keep your swaddled baby right by your bed, in a bassinet, crib, or cosleeper. Don't bring her into your bed for at least the first six months.

Make sure the device has a wide base (so it's not easy to knock over). It should also have a firm mattress with a snug fit and the sides should be at least fifteen inches high (measured from the mattress base).

If you choose a crib, make sure the crib is safe and properly assembled. (For guidance, visit the US Consumer Product Safety Commission's website.)

A cosleeper combines the cozy convenience of bed-sharing with the safety of a crib. It snuggles up right next to your bed, and has a drop-down side so you can reach your baby easily for breast-feeding and to give a quick cuddle. (Just make sure that your baby is swaddled and that the cosleeper is securely attached to *your* bed to prevent accidental falls.)

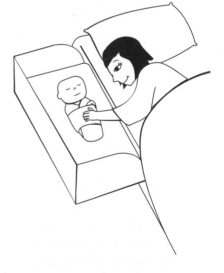

(No matter which approach you choose, make sure you follow the safety rules outlined on page 46.)

Around five or six months, many couples move their babies into a crib in another room. Babies tolerate the switch pretty easily at that age, although it's fine to wait longer. (I'll talk more about moving your baby out of your room on page 138.)

Danger Spots: Sleep Locations to Avoid

Certain sleep spots pose real risks. These include sleeping on living room furniture, sleeping sitting upright (for instance, in a car seat or infant carrier), and sleeping in poorly designed slings.

Studies from all around the world agree: sleeping on living room furniture is a *huge* risk! Scottish researchers found a sixty-seven times higher risk of SIDS among babies who were allowed to sleep on a couch. And the risk is also high for babies sleeping on recliners, armchairs, cushions, beanbag chairs, and air mattresses.

Also, the car seat is *not* a safe place for your baby to snooze in, except for little naps while you're taking a short car trip. During the first six months of life, a baby's heavy head can fall forward when she is seated, causing difficulty breathing and asphyxiation.

And how about slings? Slings are terrific. They offer a delicious flow of touch, movement, and sound, along with the continual reassurance of your scent. On top of that, they leave your hands free for other jobs. These simple folds of cloth are so helpful to new moms; I suspect they may have been one of the first bits of clothing ever invented.

However, babies frequently fall asleep in their

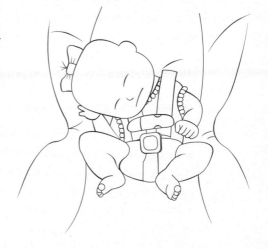

cozy slings, and that can create a real hazard. So make sure your sling:

- **Is not too deep—if your baby can sink into a little "C" position at the bottom, she is at risk for suffocation from a lack of fresh air. (Your baby should be sitting high enough so you can see her face.)**

- **Supports your baby's back so her chin doesn't fall forward and get pushed down against her chest, making it hard to breathe or cry for help.**

- **Holds your little one snug enough to protect her from falling.**

- **Has no fabric folds that can press against her nose or mouth.**

And one more sling rule: Never carry your baby in a sling when you're handling very hot food or liquids.

What about sleeping in the swing? Many swings are safer to sleep in than car seats because they can fully recline so your baby's head cannot accidentally slump forward. But only use these for babies who have difficulty sleeping without motion. (I'll have more to tell you about sleeping in the swing in the next chapter.)

As you can see, babies aren't too fussy about where they sleep. They snooze just as soundly in a plain crib as they do in the frilliest nursery. So you can paint fluffy clouds on the bedroom walls if you like, but remember that your key job is to make sure your little one sleeps *safely*. And that brings me to a controversial topic.

Bed-Sharing—Great Idea or Risky Business?

I know what I'm about to say may make me as unpopular as diaper rash with some of you. But I hope you'll bear with me, because *to bed or not to bed* is a critically important decision.

Bed-sharing is as old as the hills. From our earliest days, parents and babies have slept together for protection, warmth, and convenience. And this custom is growing in popularity; the number of bed-sharing families more than doubled between 1993 and 2000. Dr. Fern Hauck of the University of Virginia reported that 42 percent of US families bed-share at two weeks, 34 percent at three months. (The major reasons were to calm fussing, boost sleep, and make it easier to breast-feed.)

However, many tragic deaths have been reported associated with bed-sharing. For that reason, scientists have dedicated a great deal of time and effort over the past twenty years to evaluating if—and how—babies can safely bed-share. And some concerning results are emerging.

British researchers reported that most bed-sharing babies had their mouths and noses covered with bedding at some time during the night. A third of the sleeping moms also accidentally rested an arm or leg on their babies.

New Zealand infant sleep researchers, led by Sally Baddock, confirmed this risk of face covering. In a study videotaping eighty infants—forty in cribs and forty bed-sharing—the faces of the bed-sharing babies were covered a total of nearly one hour per night!

Over one hundred times, the team's camera showed babies with bedding covering their faces (usually above the eyes). Typically, the mom or baby cleared the blanket away. But a quarter of the twenty-two bed-sharers who experienced head covering still had their heads covered when they awoke in the morning. That's pretty unnerving.

Baddock also found that bed-sharing babies fed 3.7 times more often during the night, and that a quarter of the dads ended up moving out of the "family bed." And, most disturbingly, bed-sharing babies spent 66 percent of their sleep, 5.7 hours a night, *lying on their sides* (not their backs, which is a safer position). One bad-sharing baby was seen rolling all the way to the stomach.

Studies from Germany, Holland, and Scotland found that bed-sharing is associated with increased SIDS risk for babies under three to four months of age (and even older, if the parents smoked cigarettes).

On the other hand, bed-sharing Japanese babies have not been found to have a higher SIDS rate (possibly because they're sleeping on hard futons). And studies in England, Canada, and the United States found no increased bed-sharing risk with parents who are sober, attentive, and nonsmoking.

After carefully considering all the current studies, most medical groups, like the American Academy of Pediatrics and the Canadian Pediatric Society, have issued recommendations against bed-sharing with young infants. And I agree.

While I love bed-sharing with *older* children, I am too nervous to recommend it during the first four to six months (or for the first year, if you have any of the risk factors mentioned below).

I believe the best approach is to have your baby sleep *right next to your bed* in a bassinet, crib, or cosleeper . . . but not *in* your bed. You'll be able to easily nurse and comfort her, and you'll sleep better knowing that you've done everything possible to keep your precious baby as safe as humanly possible.

MAKING BED-SHARING SAFER

If, despite the concerns, you do decide to bed-share, you'll want to do everything possible to reduce the hazards. These tips can help *stack the deck* in your baby's favor and significantly lower the risks:

SAFE BED

Don't sleep on a waterbed, air mattress, or living room furniture.

Be sure there are no spaces between the mattress and the wall, bed frame, or headboard that could trap your baby's head.

SAFE BEDDING

Use only a sheet on your bed—no pillow, duvet, bumpers, stuffed animals, or positioners.

If your room is cold, dress your baby comfortably, but avoid overheating. (Touch his ears and nose; they should feel neither cold nor hot.)

SAFE BEDMATES

Don't let your baby share a bed with a smoker, pet, sibling, or someone who is obese or profoundly tired.

Keep your baby next to one parent, not between both of you.

Never use alcohol or drugs (including antihistamines) that can reduce your ability to sense your baby and react to his needs.

SAFE BABY

Always place your baby on his back.

Breast-feed if you can.

Offer a bedtime pacifier.

Don't bed-share with a preemie or a low-birth-weight baby.

SAFE ROOM

Keep the temperature between 66 and 72°F (19°C–22°C).

Ventilate your room well.

Don't use candles, incense, or a wood fire.

SAFE SWADDLING

Snugly wrap your baby in a large, light blanket to help keep him from accidentally rolling over or worming his way against the wall during sleep.

Finally, remind all family members, babysitters, and other caregivers about the importance of putting your baby to sleep on his back and all the other sleep safety rules.

Five More *Ounces of Prevention*

Here are five more tips for keeping your sleeping baby safe:

- Never leave your infant alone on an adult bed. Even two-week-olds can roll or inch their way off.

- Install smoke alarms. If you already have them, check to make sure they work.

- Install a carbon monoxide detector in the hallway near your bedrooms.

- Store an easy-to-grab fire extinguisher on each floor.

- Make an escape plan in case of an emergency (like a fire). If you live high above the ground, keep a rope ladder and a fire evacuation hood on hand.

After you install your alarms and buy your extinguishers, give your insurance company a call. They should give you a substantial discount for taking all these precautions.

Protecting Your Baby from SIDS and Suffocation

SIDS (sudden infant death syndrome) is the leading cause of death in babies between one and twelve months of age. Its peak incidence is between two and four months of age, with 90 percent of cases occurring before six months (as shown on the following graph). SIDS is not a topic anyone wants to think about—but thankfully, there are many ways to reduce your baby's SIDS risk.

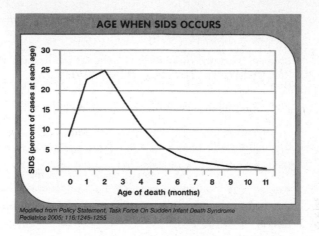

AGE WHEN SIDS OCCURS

Modified from Policy Statement, Task Force On Sudden Infant Death Syndrome
Pediatrics 2005; 116:1245-1255

The most important step is to *always place your baby on the back*!
(Interestingly, doctors used to insist that babies sleep on their
stomachs. We worried that back-sleeping babies might choke
on their spit-up. Today we know that back-sleeping babies *don't*
choke on spit-up, they just turn their faces to the side.)

Back sleeping immediately lowers a baby's risk. That's why, in
1994, doctors launched an ambitious "Back to Sleep" SIDS prevention campaign. The success was extraordinary. Within ten years,
SIDS deaths dropped by 50–80 percent . . . around the world!

Some parents resist the back position because their babies
sleep better on the stomach. But fortunately, swaddled babies
sleep just as well on the back as unswaddled babies sleep in the
riskier tummy position.

Here are the other key steps to protect against SIDS and suffocation:

- **Breast-feed at least six months if you can. (This cuts SIDS
  risk by half.)**

- **Swaddle for all naps and nights.**

- **Use a pacifier at bedtime. Formula-fed babies can start
  using a pacifier at birth, but if your baby is breast-fed, wait**

until the nursing is well established (usually one to four weeks).

- Sleep in the same room as your baby for the first six months.

- Don't bed-share with your baby for at least the first four months (and if you do it after that, make sure you do so safely).

- Strengthen your baby's neck and back with tummy exercises. (I'll talk more about this later in this chapter.)

- Avoid overheating (don't overdress her or cover her head; use thin swaddling blankets; keep the room temperature at 66°F–72°F or 19–22°C).

- Avoid soft, bulky bedding (including duvets, pillows, bumpers, stuffed animals, positioners, and lambskins).

- Avoid soft crib mattresses (including those made of feathers, memory foam, or natural fiber [treebark], and waterbeds).

- Don't place your baby to sleep on an unsafe surface (including a recliner, sofa, armchair, or beanbag chair).

- Have a smoke-free house. (Don't smoke or allow others to do so. Avoid using woodstoves, incense, scented candles, and fireplaces, if possible.)

- Don't let your baby sleep sitting up in a car seat, infant carrier, or *upright* swing, especially if she's premature or developmentally delayed. (And always ask your doctor. Only use a fully reclined swing as described on page 78.)

- Avoid cribs with missing slats, net siding, or a space between the mattress and side wall where your baby's head can be trapped.

- Don't let your baby sleep at a friend's house unless you're sure it's safe.

- Make sure your baby has received all her routine immunizations.

Unfortunately, even if you follow every rule *to the letter*, there's no guarantee of preventing SIDS. But you can be comforted by the fact that most SIDS victims have two or more risk factors. So doing everything you can will *definitely* make your baby safer.

The Baby Workout—Top Tummy Time Exercises

Routinely putting a baby to sleep on the stomach raises her risk of SIDS about fourfold. But SIDS risk jumps even higher (eight- to thirty-seven-fold) when young babies (under four months) are put to sleep on the back . . . *but accidentally roll to the stomach.*

Of course, sooner or later, your baby *will* roll onto her stomach during sleep. So what should you do to protect her? Here are some tips:

> For at least the first four months, always put your baby to sleep snugly swaddled with white noise playing nearby (see page 66). The sound will keep her calmer (less likely to fidget and roll), and the swaddling will make it harder for her to flip over.

> If your baby is less than four months old and can roll despite the swaddling and white noise, ask your doctor if she can sleep in a *fully reclined* swing (swinging, swaddled, and securely belted in) with the white noise continuing. (After she passes four months and is out of the swaddling, you won't need to worry about her flipping onto her stomach anymore. By then she will be able to push up, move her head, and roll herself back to her back.)

Once your baby reaches one month, begin daily exercises to strengthen her neck and back. That will help her develop the ability to move her face out of a blanket or mattress in case she accidentally rolls to the stomach.

Once or twice a day, hold your baby upright in your arms with her head resting on your shoulder and her belly against your upper chest. Allow her to practice lifting her head, as you gently support her neck and head with your hand.

Place your baby with her tummy and *face down* on a sheet to give her practice moving her head and getting her nose and mouth free. (Supervise her closely, and *never* leave her alone on her stomach.) The first few times, you may need to help by lifting her head a tiny bit and showing her how to swing her face to the side.

When your infant is two to three months old, place your hand under her chest during the tummy exercise to lift her a tiny bit and help her start learning how to use her arms to push up.

These exercises will teach her how to free her face by arching her back and lifting her head, in case she accidentally flips over in sleep.

Can Swaddling Reduce SIDS and Suffocation?

This is a good question, and the answer isn't absolutely clear yet— but so far it appears to be yes.

Two large studies found that swaddled, back-sleeping babies actually had about 30 percent *less* SIDS risk.

Some experts worry that swaddling might cause such deep sleep that a baby could forget to breathe, or that it might cause overheating, which can also raise SIDS risk. Fortunately, the results of studies investigating these issues are reassuring.

First, although swaddled babies sleep longer, *they don't sleep deeper*. Studies show they arouse from sleep just as easily as unwrapped babies . . . or even more easily.

And several studies show that correct swaddling helps babies keep a nice normal body temperature. They don't get overheated unless their heads are covered, they're overdressed, or the room is hot.

A careful review of all swaddling research shows that *correct* swaddling likely *prevents* sleep deaths (which is one reason the American Academy of Pediatrics recommends swaddling in their books and web articles).

However, the key word here is . . . *correct*.

Think of swaddling like car seat safety. Car seats save lives, but they can create problems if they're not installed correctly. Similarly, parents need instruction on how to swaddle safely! (I'll review that in the next chapter.)

There are several ways correct swaddling may reduce SIDS and suffocation. It may:

- **Improve sleep (reducing a parent's temptation to bed-share or to place her baby to sleep on the stomach)**
- **Reduce the risk a baby will accidentally roll onto her stomach**
- **Prolong breast-feeding (many moms give up nursing because they're so exhausted**
- **Reduce the chance that a weary parent might accidentally fall asleep with her baby on a sofa**

This threat of accidental suffocation is of increasing concern. The US Centers for Disease Control estimates that since 1994, these deaths are up 400 percent.

Why are they going up? One major reason is that exhausted parents are increasingly falling asleep with their babies in bed or on a couch, bed, or recliner. This poses two significant risks:

- **A baby may accidentally roll to her stomach and suffocate on a cushion or thick blanket.**

- A parent may be so deeply asleep that her arm may flop over the baby, and yet she may be too tired to realize the baby is struggling.

A correctly swaddled baby, sound asleep on her back in a cool room, is a safe and happy baby. Swaddling allows *everyone* to sleep better and may save many lives.

Now, Finally—on to the Fun Stuff!

I know we've talked about some scary stuff in this chapter. But if you take all the precautions I've outlined, the chance of any of this happening is very, very low.

And with all the serious stuff out of the way, it's time to head for the fun part! In the next chapter, you'll learn how to use the *calming reflex* and 5 S's to calm even the fussiest babies fast and to train your baby to sleep an extra one to two hours every night.

Does sleep training a brand-new baby sound too good to be true? Well, I'll show you how to make this miracle happen.

Crib Notes:
Reviewing the *Happiest Baby* Way

- Teach your new baby good, easy to do sleep cues and to avoid accidentally getting her hooked on labor-intensive cues (like always being rocked to sleep).

- Contrary to the opinion of most experts, babies can be trained to sleep better . . . in the first weeks of life.

- You can do many things to dramatically reduce your baby's risk of SIDS and suffocation . . . including *correct* swaddling.

## CHAPTER THREE

Helping Your Baby Fall Asleep: Birth to Three Months

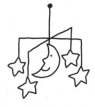

KEY POINTS:

★ Want a little more sleep? The right baby sleep cues are your *key* to success.

★ Older kids may get bratty if overindulged, but it's impossible to spoil a newborn.

★ The road to great sleep (for everyone!) starts with understanding why babies need a *fourth trimester* of cuddling and care.

★ Turning on your baby's amazing *calming reflex* is easy once you can do the *5 S's* (swaddle, side/

stomach position, shush, swing, suck) correctly
and in combination.

★ **Does putting your baby on a schedule make sense?
Only if you're flexible!**

★ **Multiples and preemies have special issues . . . but
a few tricks can help them sleep more soundly.**

People who say they sleep like a baby usually don't have one.
—Leo J. Burke

Cue the Sandman!

For sleep-deprived new parents, a good night's rest may feel like
the gold at the end of the rainbow . . . seemingly possible, yet
maddeningly out of reach.

Our babies snooze in such short dribs and drabs, it's hard for
us to get any solid sleep. And even if your baby dozes for three
hours, by the time you fall asleep you'll probably only clock in two
good hours.

This may be survivable for a few nights, but as the weeks pass,
sleep deprivation can cause profound exhaustion and can trigger
a host of serious problems—from marital struggles to depression
to car accidents to obesity.

So what's the solution?

Many experts tell new parents to just "wait it out." But I've
found that most babies—even newborns—can learn to sleep
longer . . . and at a time that's more convenient for the family.

As unlikely as it sounds, even babies newly home from the hospital can be taught to sleep better. In fact, shaping your baby's
sleep is usually pretty easy to do . . . with the right *sleep cues*.

If you've been a follower of my *Happiest Baby* classes or DVD,
you already know some of the cues I recommend, but in these
chapters, you'll learn how to use these methods—and a few new
Happiest Baby way techniques—specifically to prevent sleep problems and to make good sleep even better.

It All Starts with Sleep Cues

As I've mentioned, we all have sleep habits. I personally hate the foam pillows used in most hotels, but give me a nice feather pillow—and some *rain on the roof* white noise—and I'm out like a light. The point is . . . we're all creatures of habit.

Some parents worry that using comforting cuddling or white noise CDs will risk creating an *addiction* or "bad" habits. So what distinguishes *good* sleep cues from *bad* sleep crutches?

Simple: Good cues help your baby fall asleep fast—and stay asleep longer—yet they're easy to use, require little effort on your part, and are easy to wean.

Bad sleep cues, on the other hand, may get your baby to sleep, but they're inconvenient, very demanding on you, and difficult to wean.

For example, if your baby needs thirty minutes of bottom-patting each time he rouses or demands that only Mommy can put him to sleep (and screams if Daddy tries to step in), I think it's pretty clear you're looking at a bad sleep cue.

During the first few months, the best sleep cues are those that mimic the calming sensations of the womb. What are those sensations? To find out, let's take a trip back in time . . . to the week before your baby's birth.

Is Pregnancy Too Short? The Missing Fourth Trimester

I know what you're thinking: *Are you kidding? Too short?!* For many moms, the last month of pregnancy seemed interminable. Heartburn, puffy ankles, stretch marks, and peeing every two hours can take all the shine off that pregnancy glow.

But while you couldn't wait to finally hold your baby in your arms, your baby would definitely have voted for a few extra months inside if you had given her the choice.

Remember—your baby's brain was so big that you had to "evict" her after nine months, even though she was still smushy, mushy, and very immature. As a result, she isn't quite ready for the big, bad outside world.

After three months, your little one will be skilled at smiling, cooing, and having little conversations with you (and the birdies outside). But for the first months, you should think of her like a fetus . . . *outside the womb.*

In fact, grandmas, nurses, and nannies who are gifted baby calmers all have one talent in common: they're really good at mimicking a baby's life in the womb.

To be a good *womb impersonator,* you first need to know: "What was it like in there?" Warm? Sure. Dark? Actually, fetuses see soft red light as the rays of the sun pass through your outer skin and muscle. Quiet and still? No way!

Before birth, fetuses are lavished with rhythmic sensations: the caress of velvet-soft walls, lots of jiggly motion, and loud whooshing from blood pulsing through the uterine arteries (BTW, they don't hear your heart beat).

For centuries, smart moms have known that a little rocking and rolling soothes babies. But only recently have we realized *why* imitating the womb works so well . . . it triggers the *calming reflex.*

The Happiest Baby Way

THE GREAT AMERICAN MYTH—YOU CAN SPOIL A BABY

In a few months, your baby will start to use crying to manipulate you. But for now, you actually *want* him to learn that whenever he cries, you'll come.

Your predictable support during these early months nurtures your infant's trust and security. And that trust will become the solid foundation for *all* his loving relationships, throughout the rest of his life.

Don't worry if you're stuck on the phone when your baby launches into a tirade. A minute of crying doesn't cause mental trauma. But studies show that repeatedly ignored cries *are* a real stress that can undermine an infant's core confidence. This confidence—what child experts call *attachment*—is the glue that holds good families together.

Think of it this way: when friends ignore your calls, you may try again—but if you're repeatedly spurned, you'll eventually stop reaching out. Similarly, a baby whose smiles and coos go unreturned will initially try harder to get attention—but if he continues to get no reaction, he'll soon stop reaching out and feel rejected and alone.

But when you meet your baby's needs—dozens of times a day—with comforting arms or sips of warm, sweet milk, he'll feel, "This is a really great place. Whenever I need something, it just comes . . . it's like magic! I can really trust these people."

After nine to twelve months, it will become important to start teaching your child the meaning of limits and following the rules. (*"You can cry for an hour . . . there's no way I'm gonna let you hold the scissors!"*) But right now, your baby doesn't need discipline. What he needs is an unshakable faith that he's precious, protected, and respected. This nurturing is as critical to his growing spirit as milk is to his developing body.

So be patient! Over the coming weeks and months, you're going to gently teach your baby he is loved. You can start right away by using the best cues that help him drift off to sleep and give him the confidence to slumber securely and fall back to sleep when he wakens. However, you'll do it in easy baby steps, so his faith in you grows and grows.

The *Calming Reflex*—Nature's Off Switch for Crying and On Switch for Sleep

Clever parents have invented many ways to mimic the womb, from vacuuming to cruising deserted streets at 3 A.M. in a Volvo, hitting every pothole they see. But only recently have we discovered what imitating the womb actually does that soothes babies: it triggers a powerful neurological response called the *calming reflex*.

Okay, a word about reflexes. They're automatic behaviors that never have to be learned because they're built into our brains. For example, whether you're a newborn or a ninety-year-old, when the doctor whacks your knee with a little hammer, your foot jumps out. And amazingly, even if she whacks your knee correctly a thousand times, your foot will dutifully pop out every time!

It may look like magic, but it's really just basic physiology.

However, if your doctor smacks your knee an inch too low or a bit too softly, *absolutely nothing happens!* That's because reflexes are only turned on when they're triggered exactly right.

The *5 S*'s—Five Ways to Turn On the *Calming Reflex*

As with the knee reflex, the *calming reflex* only gets turned on when we imitate womb sensations accurately. As those who have been exposed to the *Happiest Baby* DVD or book already know, the five steps that activate the *calming reflex*—the five steps of perfect *wombihood*—are called the 5 S's.

Here's a review of these steps. After you read about the correct way to do them, I'll describe exactly how to combine these precious tools into a perfect sleepy-time ritual.

The *5 S*'s are:

1. **SWADDLING**—snug wrapping with the arms down.

2. **SIDE/STOMACH**—placing your baby on the stomach or on the side rolled toward the stomach. (Note: Never leave your

baby on the side or stomach. This position is *only* safe when your baby is in your arms!)

3. SHUSHING—strong, rumbly white noise.

4. SWINGING—rhythmic motion, from slow rocking to fast, tiny jiggling.

5. SUCKING—sucking on your nipple, a clean finger, a bottle, or a pacifier.

The 5 S's are the birthday present your baby really wants from you. Babies don't just *enjoy* the S's, they're literally transported by them into a feeling of irresistible calm and serenity. Use the 5 S's whenever your little kitten is fussy and whenever you want her to sleep.

But to succeed with the 5 S's you need to use them correctly. Swaddle too loosely, and your baby will struggle even harder. Shush too softly, and her yelps will continue as if you were totally silent. And once your baby calms, you'll need to do a reduced version of the S's—swaddling plus a bit quieter sound and slower swinging—to keep the reflex turned on.

Amazingly, the 5 S's even comfort adults (think of ocean sounds, rocking in a hammock, or relaxing in a warm bath). But womb rhythms aren't a cure-all. If your child is hungry or her ear hurts, the S's may momentarily calm the crying, but she'll soon start back with her complaints.

A study in Boulder, Colorado, showed this clearly. Public health nurses gave *The Happiest Baby* DVD and CD of white noise, plus a large swaddling blanket, to forty-two families with fussy babies. Within days, the 5 S's had helped forty-one of the infants stay calmer and sleep better (even babies withdrawing from drugs). Interestingly, the only baby who wasn't helped was soon diagnosed with an ear infection. And as soon as that was treated, the 5 S's settled his daily fussing, too.

The key to the *calming* reflex is finding your baby's favorite mix of the S's. So let's review them one at a time. (You can find a detailed demonstration and discussion of the *calming reflex* and 5 S's in *The Happiest Baby* DVD or digital download.)

The First "S": Swaddling—A Feeling of Pure "Wrap"ture

After weeks of constant crying and meager sleeping, Ann and Marty were going crazy. Nothing was working for their unhappy seven-week-old, Madison.

"We'd heard of the 5 S's, but we already knew that Maddy hated the wrapping," Marty said. "However, we were so desperate and exhausted we decided to try it."

That evening, Ann and Marty swaddled Madison and cranked up the white noise. "As always," Marty recalled, "she fought the swaddling. But with the strong womb sound she quickly fell into sleep in Ann's arms. Ann joked that Maddy seemed like a burrito in a windstorm. But that night was no joke; Maddy slept six hours straight! In the middle of the night we fed and changed her and then she went back down for another three hours.

"Suddenly, Maddy was a star sleeper! I swear, it was as if she'd been waiting for us to learn what to do."

For your baby, swaddling is the most normal thing in the world! The womb kept your precious little one wrapped in a tight ball for months. But after birth, the sudden absence of your uterine walls allows her to spin her arms like windmills, whack herself in the face . . . and wake up the whole household.

Swaddling is the *cornerstone* of calming and sleep because it keeps babies from waking with every twitch and startle. For many babies, swaddling doesn't instantly cause calming, but it does stop them from flailing. And once you add to the swaddling one or two (or three) of the other S's, the *calming reflex* suddenly switches on and helps them slide into delicious sleep. (And swaddling helps them sleep longer and safer, too.)

In truth, many babies initially fight the wrap. They struggle and scream and seem to hate it. (Certainly *we* wouldn't want to be swaddled.) But think about it. Wouldn't you also hate living in a womb for nine months or drinking milk for breakfast, lunch, and dinner? Yet I bet your baby is quite happy with that. And I also bet she'll be happy with swaddling if you stick with it . . . and combine it with a few more well-done S's.

There are many premade swaddlers on the market today, but the best method to use to swaddle your baby in a flat blanket is the *D-U-D-U* (down-up-down-up) wrap (you can see several demonstrations of this on *The Happiest Baby* DVD).

To get started:

- **Place the blanket on the bed like a diamond, with a point at the top.**

- **Fold the top corner down a bit.**

- **Place your baby's neck right over the top edge of the blanket.**

Now comes the DUDU wrap:

DOWN: With your baby's right arm straight against her side, bring the blanket *down* from her right shoulder and pull it *very* tightly across her body. (It should look like half of a V-neck sweater.) Grab the top edge of the blanket next to her *unwrapped* left shoulder and pull it so the fabric is snug around her right arm.

UP: Straighten her left arm and bring the bottom corner straight *up* to cover the arm (place the bottom blanket point right on her left shoulder). *Her legs should easily be able to bend and open at the hips,* but her arms must be straight and snug.

DOWN: Grab the blanket three inches from the left shoulder, pull the blanket taut, and bring it *down*—but only a smidge—and hold it against the center of her chest.

UP: As your left hand keeps that fold on her chest, grab the last free blanket corner (on your baby's left side) and pull it slightly *up* and across her lower chest. Wrap it around her body like a tight belt, holding her forearms firmly against her sides.

Here are a few more key tips for award-winning—and safe— wrapping:

- **Use a big (44-inch) square blanket or a premade swaddler.**
- **Your swaddled baby should only sleep on the back!**
- **Make sure she isn't too hot. Her ears should be warm, not hot and red, and her neck shouldn't be sweaty. (Don't cover your baby's head during sleep unless your doctor tells you to do so.)**
- **Only swaddle during naps, nights, and fussy periods (not twenty-four hours a day!).**

If your baby keeps struggling against the wrap or breaking out, double-check to make sure that your swaddling is snug and that your blanket is big enough.

Finally, I recommend you swaddle during all naps and night-time for *at least* four months, although some infants need the wrapping for several more months. (You can learn when and how to wean swaddling on page 179.)

Shivers and Twitches

A newborn's brain is so immature that it has a hard time controlling that little body. Sometimes, babies want to suck a finger but end up poking a thumb in their eye instead of their mouth. And sometimes their chins tremble, even though they're not cold or nervous.

Why? Because it takes a baby's brain a few months to build little fat layers around each brain cell to insulate the nerves. And until that happens the nerves have a tendency to short-circuit.

This is why swaddling a baby with the arms out doesn't work well. It doesn't suppress the sudden shivers, twitches, and startles that wake babies up and start them crying.

....

CLEARING THE AIR: DISPELLING SOME MYTHS ABOUT
SWADDLING

Swaddling is the foundation of safe, happy baby sleep. Nevertheless, there's a bit of misinformation about this ancient parenting technique swirling around the Internet. So let me set the record straight and clear up some of the most common questions you'll hear about swaddling.

"Does swaddling hurt a baby's hips?"

Antiquated wrapping techniques (with the knees and hips kept rigidly straight, or legs tightly bound with cloths or ropes) can hurt a baby's hips (developmental dysplasia of the hip, or DDH). But no study shows that this is a risk with our modern style of swaddling. The key is to make sure the hips have enough room to fully move.

The International Hip Dysplasia Institute says that swaddling is safe as long as the knees can flex and the hips can flex and open up easily.

"Should I stop swaddling once my baby can roll over?"

After a month or two, your baby may start rolling to her stomach. Swaddling usually makes it harder to roll. But what if she can roll even when she's fully swaddled?

Some doctors suggest stopping swaddling at that point for safety reasons. But many mobile babies still need swaddling to help them sleep. And besides, unwrapped babies can roll to the riskier tummy position . . . *even more easily!*

Fortunately, you can do two things to keep your wrapped baby from flipping over:

- **Use white noise all night. This will make her less fidgety and therefore less likely to roll.**

- **Place her—swaddled—in a *fully reclined* swing, secured in place with the harness or belt around her belly and between her legs. (Do not allow your baby to sit too upright. Her heavy head may fall forward and dangerously block her breathing.) Always ask your doctor if your baby is ready to sleep in the swing.**

"Will swaddling keep my baby from learning to self-soothe by sucking her fingers?"

In the womb, babies suck their thumbs because the snug uterine walls keep their hands right next to their mouth. But after birth, your baby's hands can fly all over the place when she tries to suck her fingers—sometimes in the mouth, sometimes up the nose, sometimes in the eye!

You can give your cherub some unwrapped time every day to practice finger sucking . . . but you don't want her whacking herself and waking from sleep. I recommend that during naps and nights you meet her sucking drive with a pacifier and keep her hands swaddled, for at least the first four months.

"Can swaddling undermine breast-feeding?"

Maternal exhaustion and infant crying are terrible for nursing. They dry up milk, block letdown, reduce a mom's confidence, undermine her family's support, push women toward postpartum depression and smoking (both of which lower nursing success), increase the risk of mastitis, and lead doctors to recommend difficult elimination diets and even total weaning.

So learning how to calm a baby's crying and boost sleep can actually *boost* nursing success, not undermine it. That's why hundreds of breast-feeding clinics help nursing moms succeed by teaching them swaddling and the other S's, as part of *Happiest Baby* classes.

However, during the first week or two, some swaddled babies get so comfy we have to rouse them every two hours during the day (and four to five hours at night) to make sure they're eating enough.

You can easily check your baby is getting enough to drink: the inside of her mouth will be slippery wet, she'll pee many times a day, and her pee will be very clear, not strong and yellow.

"Do all babies need swaddling?"

Some moms tell me, "My baby sleeps fine without swaddling—so can I skip it?" If you're in this situation, you certainly don't *have to* swaddle. But there are two reasons why I'd still recommend you do it:

- **Babies sleep on their backs better when wrapped (even if they're sleeping pretty well without it).**
- **Swaddling may prevent SIDS or suffocation by keeping your baby from flipping onto her stomach.**

The Second "S": Side or Stomach—But Never for Sleep!

The back is the only safe position for sleep, but it's the worst position for stopping a baby's fussies. It makes babies feel insecure, like they're falling. For crying babies, lying on the stomach (or side, rolled toward the stomach) works the best. (Another good position is up over your shoulder.)

However, you should never leave your baby placed on the stomach because that increases the risk of SIDS or suffocation. So keep your fussy little child in your arms until she's calm and then be sure to follow the "back to sleep" rule.

The Third "S": Shushing—The Sound of Silence

For a baby, a strong *shhhuuussshh* is the sound of serenity.

It may seem counterintuitive that our tender infants would like such a rough, loud noise; certainly we wouldn't. But remember—

the sound they heard in the womb was louder than a vacuum cleaner!

So quiet rooms—that *we* find restful—actually drive babies a little crazy. After hours of silence, they often start screaming. It's as if they're begging, "Please, someone make a little noise!" And as you'll see below, it's easy to give them exactly what they want.

The Happiest Baby Way

SECRETS FOR SUCCESSFUL SHUSHING

Although most parents swaddle their babies these days, it amazes me how few use white noise. White noise works miracles with fussy babies and is an amazingly powerful cue to boost baby sleep. This special sound is as important as swaddling. It's a key tool in the *Happiest Baby* sleep approach . . . and it's simple to do!

The sound needed to turn on the *calming reflex* when a baby is crying is a rough, rumbly whooshy noise that's *as loud* as his crying. You can provide this sound simply by putting your mouth close to your baby's ear and making a strong *"Shhhhhhhhhhhhhhh."*

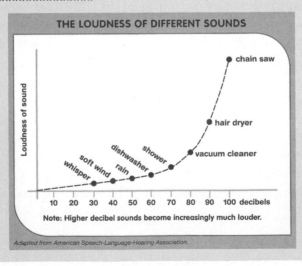

THE LOUDNESS OF DIFFERENT SOUNDS

Loudness of sound

whisper
soft wind
rain
dishwasher
shower
vacuum cleaner
hair dryer
chain saw

10 20 30 40 50 60 70 80 90 100 decibels

Note: Higher decibel sounds become increasingly much louder.

Adapted from American Speech-Language-Hearing Association.

Once your baby is calm, lower the level of your white noise to about the loudness of a shower (65–70 decibels) to keep the *calming reflex* on.

And, to help your baby doze off easily and sleep soundly, white noise is a *must*. The best white noise for sleeping mimics the sound babies hear in the womb.

As with swaddling, white noise should not be used twenty-four hours a day. You'll want to play it to calm crying episodes and during naps and nighttime sleep (start the sound quietly in the background during your sleepy-time routine, to get your sweetie ready to glide into dreamland).

After three to four months, the *calming reflex* will gradually disappear. But by then, your infant will be aware of the connection between white noise and the pleasure of sleep. "Oh yeah, I recognize that sound . . . now I'll have nice sleep." Many parents continue the white noise for years, but it's simple to wean whenever you want (more on this later).

I prefer using CDs, mobile apps, and MP3s of your baby's beloved white noise rather than sound machines. A CD is easy to use in the car (to soothe crying) and helps your child maintain good sleep—and ignore disturbing odors and lights—while you're on vacation or visiting Grandma and Grandpa. CDs and digital recordings also let you choose the exact sound and intensity that work best.

Two cautions about smartphones: They release microwave radiation so you should always put yours on *airplane mode* when you place it near your baby. And telephone and computer speakers *do not* make the best sound for babies. They make a hissy/tinny noise, not the deep, rumbly sound that best mimics the womb.

Not All White Noise Is Created Equal

Success with the *5 S*'s depends on doing a very accurate imitation of the womb. When it comes to sound, that means picking noise that's as close as possible to what unborn babies hear. And that's where the story gets interesting.

It turns out that not all white noise is created equal!

Recordings of womb sounds are harsh and hissy, but that's *not* the way they sound to your baby's ears. Amniotic fluid, thick eardrums, and middle ear fluid dampen the hissy, tinny sound of the whoosh. So, in the womb, infants actually hear a deep, thunderous rumble.

Yet most white noise machines and downloads (from ocean waves to hair dryer sounds) are high pitched. That's a problem for some babies (and parents) because our brains automatically wake up and pay attention to high-pitched sounds (think ambulance siren and smoke alarm). On the other hand, we're soothed and lulled with deeper sounds (think plane rumbling).

For this reason, our *Happiest Baby* white noise is specially engineered to reduce high-pitched sounds and amplify lower-pitched rumbling.

Your baby will love rumbly sound, but if it bothers you, try these steps to turn the noise into your new best friend:

- Play it softly in the background each evening for a week, before you start using it all night in your bedroom. That will allow your brain to get used to it.
- Put a towel or sweatshirt over your speakers to filter out even more of the high-pitched sound.
- If all else fails, you can wear a pair of good earplugs (as long as someone else can hear the baby if she cries).

How Rumbly Is the Womb? Try It Yourself

To understand what your baby heard in the womb, try this little experiment.

Run the water into your bathtub—full blast. Hear how loud and high-pitched it is? Now, when the tub is mostly full, get in the tub and dunk your head under the water. Did you notice how the sound became much more rumbling and deep?

That deeper sound is much closer to what babies hear in the womb. That's why they do best with sounds engineered to remove the high-frequency hiss. It's this rough rumble you're aiming for to comfort your baby—and to help *you* sleep better as well!

CLEARING THE AIR: DISPELLING SOME MYTHS ABOUT SHUSHING

Some parents miss out on the benefits of shushing because they're misled by myths about it. Here are the most common ones I hear.

"Does white noise numb a baby?"

Not at all. White noise is not a narcotic. It merely turns on the *calming reflex*, much like cuddling and rocking do.

"If my baby sleeps fine with just the swaddling, does he still need the womb sounds?"

Absolutely yes! The right type of white noise used during all naps and nights will help your baby sleep even better and *prevent* sleep problems . . . before they occur.

Here's why:

- White noise will help keep the *calming reflex* turned on all night, reducing night waking and stopping the fussing that can lead to rolling over.

- After you wean your baby from swaddling (at four to five months), the white noise continues to promote sleep by acting like a familiar "teddy bear" of sound. It makes her feel safe and keeps her sleeping well even though she's out of the wrap.

- White noise keeps your little mouse's sleep from being broken by outside distractions (noisy trains, cold rooms, passing headlights) *and* inside disturbances (throbbing gums, passing gas, mild hunger). That's how it helps prevent middle-of-the-night waking for the entire first year . . . and longer.

"Can white noise hurt a baby's hearing?"

Good question!

There's no evidence that shower-intensity white noise has any ill effects on a child's hearing. Remember, in the womb your baby heard much louder whooshing—24/7—for months.

The only research looking at the long-term use of white noise is a series of experiments done on baby rats at the University of San Francisco. They showed some changes in the baby rodents' hearing (their auditory discrimination), but those studies have little relevance to my white noise recommendations. For example, the rat researchers used:

- Continuous noise (without a single minute of quiet . . . day or night).

- Noise for a *very* long time (the rat equivalent of the first three years of a baby's life).

- Baby rats' hearing is based on superhigh, ultrasonic squeaks and therefore may be especially sensitive to continuous sound.

The key point to remember is that white noise is *only* for sleep and fussiness. It should be turned off for most of your baby's waking hours so her hearing can get tuned in to the normal sounds of your home and family.

"Do babies get addicted to white noise?"

If by "addicted" you mean that babies love and expect to hear noise all night, they're actually already addicted to it from all the noise they heard before being born!

But that's actually a huge bonus for you because it means you can use this great tool to boost your baby's sleep. And what's especially nice about sound is that you have total control over it, so it's easy for you to wean whenever you want (for advice on weaning white noise, see page 180).

The Fourth "S": Swinging—Rock-a-Bye Baby

Shatika called her mother in Omaha in tears. "I feel like I'm in prison!"

Shatika had given birth to Drey six weeks earlier and was having a very tough time. Drey only napped when Shatika sat on a big, inflated exercise ball bed with Drey in her arms and bounced up and down. Every time Shatika stopped, Drey would start to fuss and then begin wailing again.

Shatika felt totally demoralized. Her employer had given her three months of maternity leave, and she'd bought a whole stack of novels she'd intended to read while the baby slept. But she hadn't had time to open a single book.

Every evening, battalions of zombielike parents enter their cars and cruise the city—hitting every speed bump they can find—hoping to jiggle their babies to sleep. *Motion is the only thing that keeps these babies calm.*

Lying on a motionless bed may seem appealing to you, but to your baby it's odd and unnatural. And for the 10–20 percent of all infants who are *motion lovers*, the stillness is almost intolerable.

These kids are the real *bouncing baby boys and girls*. They usually do fine with the swaddling and rumbling sounds *for the first month or so,* but then they start fussing more and waking every two to three hours unless they're energetically bounced or danced around the room. Small, jiggly motion becomes the key step for switching on their *calming reflex.*

You'll know if you've given birth to a "bouncer." Your six-week-old loves you to *boing* up and down on the edge of the bed or hip-hop around the room when she gets whiny. Rocking chairs, slings, exercise balls, and swings are essential tools to quiet these little *movers and shakers.*

Swings have the great advantage of giving parents some freedom and giving babies the soothing motion they need throughout naps and night sleep. But the trick is to use it right.

SAFELY SOOTHING YOUR LITTLE SWINGER TO SLEEP

If your baby is one of these motion lovers, she may do better with movement for naps and nights.

As mentioned in chapter 2, sleeping in a swing is safer than sleeping in an infant car seat because the seat of the swing can *fully recline.*

You don't want your baby to sit up too straight because her heavy head might slump forward and make it hard for her to breathe. While some babies have tragically died when they were left to sleep in an upright car seat or infant seat, to date there have been no reported cases of babies choking while sleeping in a fully reclined swing.

Swings are also safer than car seats because their rhythmic motion constantly stimulates a baby's breathing.

However, if you let your baby sleep in a swing, *you must do it safely!* Here are important do's and don'ts to help you keep your swinging baby happy . . . and safe:

- **Only use a swing that reclines . . . very far back! Young babies aren't strong enough to sit up. Their necks can double over, making it very hard to breathe. The seat should** go almost all the way flat (going back halfway—45 degrees—is not good enough).

- Get your doctor's okay before using the swing. This is especially important for babies with weaker necks (those under one month of age, preemies, or with neurological problems causing rag-doll-like floppiness—what doctors call *hypotonia*).

- Make sure your swinging baby is swaddled and properly strapped in (including between the legs).

- Play rough, rumbly white noise when your baby is in the swing. The sound promotes sleep *and* stimulates breathing.

- Use the fast speed. That may seem too fast, but it is totally safe. The slow speed is just too *blah* to turn on a motion-loving baby's *calming reflex*. (As I demonstrate on the *Happiest Baby* DVD, after you deposit your fussy, swaddled baby into the swing, grab the seat and move it in quick, tiny jiggles for ten to twenty seconds to switch on the *calming reflex* and stop your baby's screams.

- Protect your baby from intruders. Leaping dogs and rambunctious toddlers can knock swings over, so never leave your swinging baby unsupervised around them. (If you have a dog, let it see the swing turned on, with a doll inside. This will allow the novelty to wear off and for you to teach it to keep away.)

CLEARING THE AIR: DISPELLING SOME MYTHS ABOUT SWINGING

Just as with swaddling and shushing, there are misperceptions about swinging . . . and these false ideas can get in the way of your baby's sleep. So let's take a minute to look at the facts.

"Are swings bad for a baby's hips or back?"

Inside the womb, babies are twisted like pretzels. Actually, newborns are as flexible as little yoga experts! So there's no concern for your baby's hips or back in the swing.

"Do swings make parents neglect their babies?"

Your baby should be in someone's arms as much as possible. But unless you have a dozen willing relatives helping you, there may not be enough arms to go around. So when you're short on helpers, a swing is a very useful tool (and it's a godsend for parents of multiples!).

Bottom line: Thinking you're a better parent because you never use a swing is like thinking you're a better cook because you never use an electric can opener.

Swing, Never Shake—Babies, Frustration, and Child Abuse

Frank felt a wave of anger blow across him like a hot wind. After weeks of his son's colicky screaming, he got so angry he punched his hand right through the door!

"I was just so frustrated and exhausted," he said almost breaking down. "I'd never hurt my boy, but for the first time in my life I understood how a parent could be driven to such desperation."

Calming a fussy baby feels great. But when everything we do fails, the frustration can push even a loving parent into the dark abyss of child abuse.

Remember, your baby's cry can be as loud as a power lawn mower—six inches from your ear! This can trigger an internal *red alert,* making your heart pound and your skin jump. These sharp screams can break a parent's confidence and overwhelm someone who's also feeling crushed by fatigue, money stress, family fights, or past abuse.

Shaken baby syndrome (SBS) is a tragically common type of abuse, affecting thousands of babies each year. It occurs when a baby's head is whipped back and forth or hit against a surface. The average victim's age is three and a half months. About 25 percent of severely shaken babies die, and up to 80 percent of the survivors suffer brain damage. *And the top trigger is . . . infant crying.*

The very idea of SBS makes some parents afraid to even jiggle their babies at all. But please be assured . . . there's a huge, huge difference between shaking and swinging.

Shaking is rough and violent. A baby's heavy head snaps back and forth, banging the brain against the hard walls of the skull, bruising and tearing the delicate tissues. The American Academy of Pediatrics notes, "The act of shaking leading to shaken baby syndrome is so violent that individuals observing it would recognize it as dangerous and likely to kill the child."

Swinging isn't like that *at all*. The jiggling motions I recommend are fast and *tiny*. They mimic what your baby experienced in the womb every day, as you walked, climbed stairs, or exercised. The movement should be *no more than one inch back and forth*. Doing this makes the head shimmy, like Jell-O on a plate, but inside the brain stays safe, barely moving.

Not only is swinging like this perfectly safe, but jiggling is such a potent baby calming tool that it can keep frustrated parents from reaching the boiling point of abusive desperation. That's why several public health programs teach this (and the other *5 S*'s) to parents to *prevent* SBS.

Nevertheless, *never* shake (or even jiggle) your baby when you're angry!

If you're at the end of your patience, put your crying baby down and take a break. Vent your stress by yelling into a pillow or punching the sofa. And seek help from your spouse, your family, a friend, or a crisis hotline. The National Child Abuse Hotline, 1–800 4-A-CHILD (1–800–422–4453), is open all day, every day.

The Fifth "S": Sucking—The Icing on the Cake

Sucking is the fifth S, but that doesn't mean you have to do it last. In fact, picking up your baby and offering milk will probably be your first S, much of the time.

Sucking and sweet warm milk not only make your baby's stomach full and happy; they also boost endorphins (the body's natural opium) in his brain, provide a flood of sleep-inducing tryptophan, and, of course, trigger the *calming reflex*. Ahhh . . . what delight!

If you're nursing, you'll want to give your newborn plenty of suckling at the breast and you should avoid rubber nipples (especially bottles!) until your baby is nursing well—usually one to four weeks.

Each gulp of milk will reward your new baby's good efforts and improve his skill, so he sucks the nipple instead of biting it. But if you have any trouble nursing, speak with your doctor, a lactation consultant, or a La Leche League leader to help you figure out what's needed to get your nursing back on track.

WHAT ABOUT PACIS?

As I noted earlier, the American Academy of Pediatrics recommends that babies fall asleep at night sucking a pacifier. That's because studies show that this can reduce the risk of SIDS.

No one really knows why bedtime paci sucking protects against SIDS (which usually occurs many hours into sleep). But it seems like it does. (By the way, if the paci pops out during the night, you don't have to put it back in.)

When you offer a pacifier, be sure to do it safely. Here's how:

- **Buy clear silicone pacifiers instead of yellow rubber ones. The yellow rubber gets sticky and deteriorates after a while and may release tiny amounts of an unhealthy chemical residue.**

- **Never dip a pacifier into syrup or honey. This can cause infant botulism, a potentially fatal disease.**

- Wash the pacifier with soap and water every day. In one study, 80 percent of pacifiers had a little film of yeast or bacteria growing on them. Also, don't put the paci in your mouth to clean it. You might accidentally pass along a cold or even herpes.
- Never hang a pacifier around your baby's neck. Strings may get tightly wrapped around the fingers (cutting off circulation) or around the neck (causing choking).

Reverse psychology: A trick for teaching your reluctant baby to take a paci

If your baby resists taking the paci try offering it when she relaxes, towards the end of a feed. But if that fails, try reverse psychology.

I asked Denise if her son, Aidan, liked pacifiers. She laughed and emptied a little sack onto the kitchen table. Six different pacifiers scattered across the tabletop, looking like a collection of lunar rocks. "He's rejected every single one!" she said with a tone of resignation.

I suggested that Denise try a different approach: rather than pushing the pacifier in every time he popped it out, she should pull on it a little every time he gave it a little suck!

Toward the end of a nursing—when Aidan relaxed and his sucking slowed—Denise tried this trick; removing her breast and immediately sliding in the paci (like a classic "bait-and-switch"). When it was snugly in his mouth, she would wait for him to suck on it . . . then she would pull it back a smidge, like testing if a fish is on the line. He responded by sucking harder.

For the next ten minutes, Denise played this little game of "reverse psychology" with Aidan to teach him how to keep the pacifier in his mouth. She repeated this exercise a few times a day and within three days Aidan took the pacifier easily.

Some babies are little sucking machines! (This is a genetic trait that runs in families.)

But even if your baby is lukewarm about sucking a pacifier—or gets confused and pushes it out instead of sucking it in—you can probably persuade her to like it by practicing the simple technique I used with Aidan. (This works best before a baby turns six weeks old.)

This bit of reverse psychology is based on our natural feeling that "what's in my mouth belongs to me." Eventually, trying to remove the nipple will become like prying a toy from a two-year-old; the harder you pull, the more she'll resist.

Clearing the air: Addressing one common concern about sucking

Nursing mothers often worry: "Will my baby's sucking on a pacifier interfere with her nursing?"

Many babies can successfully suck on anything you put in their mouth. But some nursing babies get "nipple confusion" if they're also given bottles or pacifiers before they fully get the hang of breast-feeding. That's because to get milk, breast-fed babies have to *relax the mouth* and open widely, while bottle-fed babies have to mash down on the nipple to get the formula or to slow its flow . . . and you can imagine how that *jaw clamp* feels on your nipple!

So if you're breast-feeding, it's best to avoid all bottles until your baby is nursing well, usually two to three weeks. (Of course, if she's sick and needs to take a bottle, that's a different story.)

It's also best to also avoid pacifiers until the nursing is well established, but research increasingly shows that most babies can suck on pacis without getting nipple confusion.

Putting It All Together: Creating a Sleeptime Routine for Your Infant

With the 5 S's you're now fully armed to trigger your baby's *calming reflex* anywhere, anytime to soothe crying *and* to speed slumber. So now it's time to put all this information together to help your baby at each stage of the first few months.

Soothing Your Sweetie During the First Days

During the first week or two, most babies are supercomfy with just the swaddle and sucking. But, once you're home, I recommend you also add white noise. Remember, silence is weird and unsettling to babies who heard loud whooshing 24/7 before birth.

Adding 5 S's Over the Next Three Months

As the weeks pass, in addition to the swaddling, white noise, and sucking (this is when you might add the pacifier), your baby may develop the need for jiggly motion for calming or for sleep. Ask your pediatrician's permission for her to be in a *fully reclined* swing. (Remember to always follow the tips on safe swinging on page 78.)

As you add sleep cues, don't fret about how you'll wean them when your angel is old enough to self-soothe without them. It will be simple, and I'll teach you all about it in the chapters to come.

Experiment a little, and see what combination of S's works best for you and your little one. (Trust me . . . she'll let you know!) Here's a chart to review the general approach.

Which *S*'s to Use When

In the hospital	**Sucking and swaddling**
The first week or two	**Sucking, swaddling, and white noise**
The next several months	**Sucking, swaddling, white noise, swinging (fully reclined), and a pacifier**
At all three stages	**Calm your baby by putting her on her tummy when you're holding her . . . but always put her on her back to sleep!**

Tech Support: Finding Help If the 5 *S*'s Aren't Working

Of course, each baby is an individual and no tool works 100 percent of the time. But in my experience, when done *correctly,* the *5 S*'s calm crying and boost sleep over 90 percent of the time.

So if you're doing the *5 S*'s and your baby is still crying, first make sure you're doing each step correctly (speak to your *Happiest Baby* educator or review the demonstrations on *The Happiest Baby* DVD). But if you're sure you're doing the *S*'s right, you should call your baby's doctor to check for a medical problem (like a food allergy or an ear infection).

Calming Very Fussy Babies: Kick It Up a Notch

Soft whispers and gentle rocking are perfect for calm babies. But fretful infants need a bit more vigor to help them calm and fall asleep. This sounds as wrong as the advice to add a slimy, raw egg to a cake mix . . . yet it's every bit as true!

Think of turning on the *calming reflex* like getting someone's attention. If a person is engaged in a heated argument, you may have to tap his shoulder several times—very emphatically—just to get him to respond.

Vigor is exactly why vacuum sounds and car rides on bumpy roads calm babies. And it's why grabbing the swing seat and giving some fast—but tiny—jiggles is essential to flip on the *calming reflex* in a screaming, motion-loving baby.

(Of course, you must never shake your baby! When jiggling, always support your baby's head and neck and keep your movements to just about one inch back and forth.)

Think of baby calming as a dance . . . and your little love is leading. When he's wailing, use more intensity in your shush and jiggle. Then, as he calms, gradually reduce your effort and guide him down to a *soft landing* where he is just swaddled with white noise (as loud as a shower) and perhaps some sucking or gentle rocking.

Dads: The Kings of Calm

A nurse in Boise told me that in the middle of a neighborhood softball game, a baby started to cry in the stands. Abruptly, the third baseman called a time-out, sprinted to the bleachers, swaddled and shushed his little baby into calm, and ran back on the field, all in under a minute. She said the crowd rewarded him with a thunderous ovation.

Dads and moms bring different skills to baby care. And while men are not very good at breast-feeding, we're supergood at swaddling and baby calming. To us, the wrapping is like an engineering task.

Vigor is also another reason why dads are such good baby calmers. If moms are from "Cuddleland," dads are from "Jiggleland." While moms prefer soft singing and gentle rocking, dads confidently put enough oomph into their rumbling shushing and wiggly jiggling to reach the needed "takeoff velocity" to switch on the *calming reflex*.

And when we get really good at calming our fussy babies, we feel great pride in our skills . . . and want to meet our child's needs every chance we get!

The Happiest Baby Way

A CRAZY/SMART TIP: THE WAKE-AND-SLEEP TECHNIQUE

At this point, I'd like to share one of this book's key *Happiest Baby* suggestions. I know you may think I've lost my marbles. But humor me. This method is superimportant to improving the sleep of *everyone* in the family. It's called *wake-and-sleep*.

Many sleep experts warn that moms who lull their babies to sleep in their arms or while suckling are setting themselves up for misery. They caution that these babies won't learn to self-soothe and will scream for Mama's help every time they pop awake.

The advice may sound reasonable, but it puts parents in a terrible bind!

Yes, rocking or nursing a baby to sleep every night *will* create a sleep cue she'll expect (and demand) at every waking. But honestly, *it's totally impossible* to keep your baby from zonking out when she's in a cozy cuddle with a stomach full of warm, sweet milk.

Furthermore, it's just wrong to tell parents and caregivers *not* to cuddle their babies to sleep. There is nothing more beautiful than rocking your sleeping precious in your arms! You're not spoiling your baby when you do this, you're teaching her that you love her and she can depend on you. So feel free to caress and carry your sleeping baby for as many hours as you like; you will truly grieve the loss of this sacred intimacy once these months are over.

But here's the problem: repeatedly rocking and nursing your baby to sleep *will* create sleep problems by preventing her from learning to self-soothe.

It's confusing, huh? So what's a parent to do? Luckily, there's an easy solution to this puzzle!

When you're ready to settle your baby for the night:

1. Turn on a track of white noise (at the intensity of a shower).

2. Give a nice feeding with lots of delicious holding and rocking.

3. After the feeding, swaddle and rock your snoozing munchkin as long as you want.

BUT . . .

When you place her in the crib—swaddled and with the sound playing—*jiggle her to wake her up a tiny bit.*

After a good feed, babies act kind of *drunk* from the milk. So when you rouse your child, her eyes will open for a few seconds, but then she'll probably just slide back into slumberland.

However, if she starts crying when you wake her, pat her back (like a tom-tom drum) or give the crib a fast, one-inch jiggle for thirty seconds to reset the *calming reflex.* If she keeps fussing, pick her up to calm her . . . *but be sure to wake her* again *when you put her back down.*

I know you're probably thinking, *Are you out of your mind? There's no way I'm going to wake my sleeping baby!* But this is one of the most important tips I can teach you!

These few seconds of drowsy waking are essential for teaching your baby how to self-soothe. Practice this now and I promise you that within a few weeks, you'll get a *huge* reward: your little friend will become much better at getting herself back to sleep (as long as she's not hungry or uncomfortable).

Finding the *Happiest Baby* Class Nearest You

Thousands of *Happiest Baby* educators teach the *5 S*'s approach to baby calming and baby sleep in hospitals, clinics, and military bases across the United States and in many other nations.

Two Arizona surveys found that *before* a *Happiest Baby* class, 40 percent of pregnant couples were moderately to very worried about being able to calm their baby's screams. But *after* the class, that dropped to just 1 percent!

Through classes and home visiting programs, professionals are helping bring the benefits of baby calming and increased sleep to all parents—from suburban yuppies to jailed moms to teen dads to parents dealing with the stress of parenting a preemie, an adopted baby, or a foster newborn.

To Schedule, or Not to Schedule . . .

After your baby reaches one month, creating some order in your day through a *flexible* schedule can be helpful, especially if you live a complicated life (you have multiples, older kids, a chronic illness, parents to care for, a job outside the house, you're a single parent, etc.).

Some doctors recommend scheduling a baby's activities in an "eat, play, sleep" sequence. Their idea is get a child out of the habit of always eating to bring on sleep (the hope is that uncoupling the two will help the baby be able to fall back to sleep without a feed if she wakes at 2 A.M.).

This sounds logical . . . but it actually goes against a baby's biology.

Babies often snooze after feeds, no matter how much you prod and play with them. And before bedtime, you'll certainly want to fill your little guy's tummy right to prolong his sleep.

I think a *flexible* schedule makes more sense. For example:

- After one and a half to two hours of daytime alertness feed your lovebug and then put him to sleep. (The goal is to start the nap before sleep signs like yawning show up.)
- If the nap goes over two hours, wake your baby up. (Long naps mean less eating during the day . . . and that leads to more hunger at night.)

The key to this schedule is being flexible. If you're planning a 1 P.M. nap, but your little guy seems exhausted at 12:30, it's fine to bend the "rules." Just feed him and put him in bed early (swaddled with the white noise playing). And, if he dozed off in your arms, deposit him in the crib, gently jostle him until his eyes open . . . then let him float back into sleep (the *wake-and-sleep* technique).

If you're concerned about how much your baby is sleeping and if she's on track, just take a quick look at the sample sleep schedules in the appendix.

The Golden Moment: Put Your Baby to Sleep Before She's Exhausted

Most people think a baby's ready for slumber when her eyes get lidded and her head slumps against our shoulder. Actually, at that point she is *overtired*.

Many babies can sleep anywhere, anytime. But those with a challenging temperament or poor state control live on a tightrope. Growing weariness can suddenly tip them off-balance and send them crashing down from happy alertness to exhausted misery in a blink.

So if your well-meaning neighbor says to keep your tired baby awake during the day to boost her sleep at night, *don't do it!* This strategy may work for adults, but it usually backfires with babies, leading to bigger struggles falling into sleep . . . and staying there.

In his classic book *Healthy Sleep Habits, Happy Baby*, sleep expert

Dr. Mark Weissbluth states, "Sleep begets sleep." He's right . . . and that's why experienced parents put their babies to sleep *before* they get overtired. As shown in the sample two-month-old schedule (on page 340) during these early months, your best bet is to put your little bug in bed after one and a half to two hours of wakefulness, hopefully at—or just *before*—she shows these early signs of fatigue:

- Reduced activity, smiling, and talking (or even increased frowning!)
- Yawning
- Staring, blinking, and rubbing the eyes
- Increased fussing

Don't Give Your Baby Cappuccino at Bedtime!

Everything was going great with Lucas . . . until he turned ten days old. Out of the blue, he had two terrible days of shrieking from 5 P.M. to midnight. His mother, Liz, said, "The only thing that would get him to quiet was to hook him up to nurse. The breast quickly calmed him and he sank into sleep. But as soon as I slipped him off . . . he wailed!"

Then Liz realized: "Oh my God! It's the coffee!" On both tumultuous days, she had downed a big cup of coffee with lunch. Happily, when Liz cut out the coffee, Lucas turned back into a little lamb again.

Even a Roman mama would never feed her baby cappuccino. But that's exactly what you may accidentally be doing if you're breast-feeding and drinking coffee! Caffeine collects in your breast milk for twelve hours after you drink it, and it can rev up your baby for much of the day (it lasts in your baby's blood for *twelve to twenty-four hours*).

Besides coffee, other culprits containing caffeine (and related stimulants) include tea (iced and hot), cola, diet pills, decongestants, certain Chinese herbs, and—unfortunately—chocolate (especially dark chocolate . . . sorry!).

Multiples—Double Your Pleasure . . . If You Can Get Some Sleep

When I was growing up, twins were very unusual . . . but today it seems like *everyone* is having them.

According to the US government, about one in thirty babies are twins—the highest rate on record. Twinning rose 70 percent between 1980 and 2004. The triplet/+ birth rate climbed more than 400 percent from 1980 through 1998 but is down 24 percent from the 1998 peak.

Parents of multiples are a special club. They have shared experiences that few other people understand. Multiples are great fun—especially once they get a bit older and they become built-in playmates—but the first months can be really hard work.

The work can be especially arduous if you needed a C-section or have a fragile baby (over 50 percent of multiples are born prematurely and have a low birth weight).

As you can imagine, it can often be tough to get enough rest (or even to pee!) during the first year of your babies' lives. Rest is especially important to help you avoid depression, which is more common among moms of multiples. (More about this on page 111.)

Yet, Elizabeth Damato, from Case Western Reserve University in Ohio, found that during the first couple of months, moms of twins slept only 6.2 hours a night (6.9 hours in an entire day). And their poor husbands only clocked in a measly 5.4 hours a night (5.8 hours in an entire day)!

Here's some advice to boost your babies' sleep . . . and yours:

- Ask your pediatrician if it's okay for you to use a *fully reclined* swing to calm one baby while you attend to the other (use swings for both for your dinner break).

- Use swaddling and white noise for all naps and night sleeping (as well as fussy periods).

- Put your babies on a flexible schedule. During the first month (corrected age), keep naps under two hours and wake after four hours of night sleep to feed. The second month (corrected age), you can extend night sleep to five or six hours—and longer after that.

- If your two-month-old babies (corrected age) still can't manage four hours of continuous night sleep, ask your doctor's permission to allow them to spend all night sleeping in *fully reclined* swings.

- Feed your babies before placing them to sleep. If they fall asleep in your arms, do the quick *wake-and-sleep* technique (see page 88).

- When you feed one baby, wake the other up to eat, too. (When one wakes, unwrap the other to start getting her awake.) That helps you organize your day and improves your chance of getting sleep.

- Nap when you can!

- Get help when you can! Family, friends, and nannies can give you little breaks . . . so you don't break.

- Make sure you follow the simple advice on page 106 to keep illness out of your house.

- Since twins are at increased risk of SIDS, be sure to follow the safe sleep tips on page 53.

Last, many moms wonder if their twins should sleep in the same bassinet or in two separate ones.

A study from Durham University in England videotaped sixty pairs of twins (0–5 months old) during sleep. At one month, 60 percent were in the same sleep location; at three months, only 40 percent were together.

Of concern, the scientists found that twins sleeping side by side would occasionally lay an arm across the other's face! This caused breathing problems (because of lowered oxygen) and required the affected twin to awaken and move her face or push the arm away. (Obviously they weren't swaddled.)

So ask your doctor's advice on this one. But if you do plan to have the twins sleep together for the first few months, make sure you swaddle them snugly (perhaps in a premade baby swaddler that cannot unravel) and put them *top to tail* (see drawing). And be sure to use rumbly white noise to keep them calm and reduce wiggling.

By two or three months, it's time to separate twins into two bassinets or cribs to keep one baby from rolling onto the other.

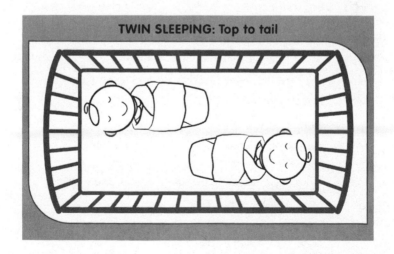

TWIN SLEEPING: Top to tail

Preemies: Helping Early Babies Get Their Sleep in Gear

If you're the parent of a preemie, you may feel shell-shocked. These babies can look so tiny and vulnerable, and the newborn intensive care unit (NICU) can be such an intimidating place.

And life with preemies continues to be tough and exhausting even when you bring your baby home. During their first weeks at home, preemies typically wake every three hours—all night. It sounds odd, but the dark stillness of home is actually jarring for babies accustomed to all the light and noise in the NICU.

Another problem that comes out of left field is a big spike in fussiness. Preemie crying typically accelerates one to two weeks after coming home. That's not just because the nurses were so gifted at calming . . . it's because preemies don't start into the normal baby fussy period until they reach their due date.

Fortunately, the *5 S*'s will give your baby some of the third-trimester cuddling she missed, *plus* an entire *fourth trimester* of soothing stimulation to keep her calm and happy.

Here's some extra advice that you might find helpful in surviving your baby's prematurity:

- During the day, give your baby lots of nursing, skin-to-skin contact, holding and rocking to keep the *calming reflex* turned on and to reduce overstimulation from the sharp noises and commotion of your home.

- Use swaddling and white noise for all naps and night sleeping, as well as fussy periods.

- If your baby still wakes every couple of hours, ask

your doctor's permission to let her sleep in a *fully reclined* swing.

- Nap when you can!

- Get help when you can!

- Keep germs and illness out of your house by following the simple advice on page 106.

A Short, Sweet, Sacred Time

Of all the times in your life, this is one of the most challenging. But as you and your baby master the ropes of family life together, there are two things I'd like you to remember:

1. This time doesn't last very long! The next few months will pass in a flash. Before you know it, you'll be sleeping through the night again.

2. This time doesn't last very long! Once this time is gone, you'll actually miss the sweet, sweet moments of holding your tiny, precious baby close to your heart and nuzzling against his soft head in the still of the night.

So hang in there . . . use the 5 S's . . . and enjoy every beautiful, crazy minute.

Crib Notes:
Reviewing *The Happiest Baby* Way

■ Babies do best with special rumbling white noise. That's what mimics the womb the best. The *right type* of white noise—for all naps and nights—is key to better sleep from day one to the first birthday . . . and well beyond!

■ Safe swaddling is the cornerstone to calming your baby and getting good sleep. And there are ways you can keep swaddling even if your little one can roll over!

■ For motion-loving babies, sleeping in a fast-moving swing is the secret to happy, restful nights.

■ Pacifiers are great for calming your baby once nursing is well established.

■ You can teach a reluctant baby to take a pacifier by using . . . *reverse psychology.*

■ A bit of vigor is essential to soothing most superfussy babies.

■ Waking your baby—after you ease her into bed— sounds nuts, but the *wake-and-sleep* technique will bring you many hours of added slumber by preventing sleep problems *before* they develop.

## CHAPTER FOUR

Stretching Your Baby's Sleep—and Yours: Birth to Three Months

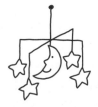

KEY POINTS:

* A happy tummy leads to peaceful sleep! In this chapter, you'll learn strategies for using feeding to help your baby snooze better and longer.

* You can prevent night waking by keeping your baby healthy—and if the sniffles strike despite your best efforts, there are steps to make sleep as comfortable as possible.

* Improve your own sleep by *just saying no* to phone calls and visitors.

★ **Postpartum depression is real, treatable . . . and
sometimes even preventable.**

*Babies are always more trouble than you thought—and
more wonderful.*

—CHARLES OSGOOD

Your Next Big Goal: Sleeping Longer!

With the help of the 5 S's, you'll be able to quickly quiet the tears
and fussing when it's time to tuck your baby in. It's a wonderful
moment when your little one serenely drifts off into sleep . . . but
as all new parents know, that's just the first hurdle.

Your next goal is to help your baby enjoy a good long stretch
of sleep. In this chapter, you'll find out how a few simple tweaks
at feeding time can translate into hours of additional sleep for
both of you. It's another pain-free, no-tears way to *sleep train* even
young babies.

And how much sleep are *you* getting during these hectic first
months? As you discovered back in chapter 1, you can't do your
best if you're deliriously sleep deprived. So later in this chapter,
I'll look at ways you and your partner can get the rest and loving
support you need . . . and I'll talk about strategies that can help to
prevent postpartum depression, a condition that can steal both
your sleep . . . and your joy.

But first . . . here's a look at the full tummy/sleep connection
and how you can use it to your advantage.

Better Nights Start with a Satisfied Tummy

It's 2 A.M. You're just sliding into sleep when you hear a squeak
from the bassinet. You say, "Oh, please . . . please . . . just another
few minutes, sweetie!" But you're already awake—waiting for the
next cry—and slumberland is fast disappearing in your rearview
mirror.

As I noted in chapter 1, your baby's sleep cycle (the full circuit from light to deep to light NREM sleep . . . plus a bit of REM) lasts only sixty minutes. So about every hour, she'll enter light sleep . . . or even briefly wake and make a short moan or squawk.

Unless she's wailing, give your little friend a few moments to soothe herself and dive right back into sleep. If she's swaddled and you're playing a rough and rumbly white noise, she should settle within thirty seconds.

However, if your princess insists you attend to her at 1 A.M. (and 3 A.M. . . . and 4 A.M.), something may be bothering her. Noises—from a snoring parent to a passing truck—can jolt her awake each time she returns to light sleep (especially if she has a sensitive temperament). But hands down, your baby's number one middle-of-the-night, snooze-shattering disturbance is *hunger*.

The Solution: Frequent Daytime Feeds

During the early months, your favorite subject may be sleep—but your baby's is definitely *food*!

In the womb, you literally fed her every single second. So it's no surprise that she needs frequent feeds to sustain her fast-paced growth. In fact, mothers in some cultures actually nurse their babies fifty to one hundred times a day! I'm not recommending that to you, but breast-fed newborns do need at least ten to twelve feedings a day. (Bottle-fed babies need six to eight.)

Is it possible to manage that and still get more than two hours sleep in a row? Yes! The key: *during the first few months* feed your little one every one to one and a half hours while he's awake during the day (if he's sleeping, let him go two hours). That should help you get a couple of back-to-back longer clumps of sleep (three to four hours) at night.

It's totally doable! And with the help of swaddling, white noise, and a *dream feed,* the night sleep should grow to five . . . six . . . then seven hours at a stretch, by three months.

Below, I'll describe how to tweak your baby's meal schedule when you're nursing. (If you're using formula, the same approach will work—just substitute a bottle.)

Breast Milk or Formula?
Choosing Your Baby's Diet

Different moms have different needs. For some, breast-feeding isn't an option, for either medical or personal reasons.

If you don't breast-feed, there are several good artificial formulas available. Formula is easy to work around your sleep schedule. (At bedtime, just put a thermos of clean warm water and a baby bottle with premeasured formula powder by your bed. Then, when your baby gets hungry, mix them together and voilà! You have fresh formula without having to totter down to the kitchen and start from scratch.) Formula also lets your partner give a feeding, allowing you to get a little catch-up sleep.

But if you *can* breast-feed, this is definitely the best way to go. Breast milk has hundreds of ingredients to build strong bodies and brains, and scores of special immune boosters (even white blood cells) to enhance immunity and prevent illness . . . and it reduces SIDS.

In addition, breast milk is always clean, warm, and available (which will save you hours of time and hundreds of dollars). And breast-feeding can also help you lose weight (your baby sucks out of you as many calories as you'd consume running three to five miles a day). Amazingly, nursing can even reduce your risk of breast and ovarian cancer!

"Sleep Training" Your Baby's Tummy

If you're nursing, it may seem like you're awake nearly all night long, but one recent study showed that nursing moms sleep just as long as formula feeders during the first few months. Another showed that nursing moms actually got forty-five minutes more sleep per night.

But even if nursing moms get a bit more total sleep each night, they definitely wake up more often. And as the months pass, their babies continue to wake for a couple of feedings a night, especially if they bed-share (unlike formula-fed babies who sleep increasingly longer stretches). It's not that your nursing baby can't go longer—she can, but only if you make an effort to teach her how.

This point was underscored by a fascinating study from the University of Illinois that raised the question, "Can we help breast-fed babies sleep better?"

The researchers told thirteen first-time moms to wake their new babies between 10 P.M. and midnight and offer them a feeding (a so-called *dream feed*). They were also told to respond to their babies' nighttime cries with a pause—a minute of loving care (reswaddling, diapering, a quick walk-and-pat)—*before* offering the baby the breast.

The results were striking.

The infants ate less at night, but more during the day (especially first thing in the morning!). Their weight gain was fine. Plus, they soon began sleeping longer—and by eight weeks, 100 percent were sleeping from midnight to 5 A.M. (compared with 23 percent of babies whose moms nursed them as usual).

So if you're nursing, here's what I recommend.

For the first month:

- **Use rumbling white noise and swaddling.**

- **Practice the *wake-and-sleep* technique (see page 88) every time your baby is put down for a nap or night sleep.**

- **Have your baby sleep right next to your bed.**

- **Feed him every one to one and a half hours during the day. (If he's napping, try not to let him go longer than two hours.)**

- **Feed just five minutes on one side and then complete the feeding on the other side. That will stimulate both breasts and still give your baby plenty of your rich hindmilk.**

- **Wake him for a *dream feed* around 11 P.M. to fill up his tummy.**

- **If your baby sleeps five hours at night, wake him for another feeding. (Some babies get so comfy they forget to wake and don't get enough milk.)**

For the next two months follow the same steps, but:

- **At night, let your baby sleep longer (he'll probably go six to seven hours, maybe even a bit longer).**
- **Pump milk from your breasts when they get too full at night. But it's best to remove only one to two ounces (pumping too much will trick your breasts into making even more milk at night!).**

Amazingly, your breasts will automatically *shift* their milk production to fit your baby's feeding schedule, making more during the day and less at night.

You'll know that your baby is getting enough to eat when:

- **He makes nice gulping noises at the start of each nursing.**
- **Your breasts feel full at feeding time (they may even leak) and much softer at the end.**
- **Your baby is happy after a feeding and not hungry again for one to two hours.**
- **His mouth is slippery wet.**
- **He has five to eight heavy, wet diapers each day, with clear or barely yellow urine.**
- **His stools are runny and seedy. (By six to twelve weeks, his poops may become thicker and golden brown, and they may only occur once or twice a day or even skip days.)**
- **His weight gain is on target. (Over the first days, your baby will lose 5 to 10 percent of his birth weight, but after that, he should gain steadily.)**

Sleep training your baby's tummy is a great way to give you and him *hours* of extra nighttime sleep.

Ahhh-Choo! Colds, Dust, and Other Sleep Stalkers

By the time their third child, Daniella, was born, Laurie and Doug felt like baby experts. So they thought it would be a piece of cake taking their two-month-old on a car ride to the Grand Canyon. Everything went fine . . . until she developed a fever and cough in Arizona. Long story short, Daniella ended up being hospitalized for three days of treatment and observation. And her cough continued to shake her little body for almost four months, waking her (and her dismayed parents) two to three times a night.

Bad colds and other bugs wreak havoc with an infant's sleep. That's because . . .

- **Infant nostrils are so tiny they easily get clogged . . . waking your baby.**
- **Coughing can cause vomiting . . . waking your baby.**
- **Diarrhea can cause a painful diaper rash . . . waking your baby.**

And the list goes on and on.

The good news is that during pregnancy, you loaded your baby up with lots of immune boosters. And if you're nursing, your babe is getting even more of these powerful defenders with every feed.

The bad news is that new babies need every bit of help they can get, because their illness-fighting ability is about on par with their golf game. So for infants, an ounce of prevention is worth a pound of cure.

Illness Prevention

Most parents are surprised to learn that most illnesses are *not* spread by droplets in the air . . . they're spread by touch. You touch the store door, then unconsciously rub your eye or nose. That's when germs sneak in and start their dastardly work.

So it's fine for you to go outside with the baby, as long as you go to a restaurant early and you steer clear of crowded places. Germs won't leap upon your little one's body; it's *contact* that's the worrisome exposure.

Here are a few ways you can beat the bugs at their own game:

- **Wash your hands . . . a lot. This really works, especially when you return home from public places. Regular soap is fine (don't use antibacterial soap, it contains harsh chemicals).**

- **Reduce visitors. Limit your guests to very close family/ friends and people who will help you cook or clean.**

- **Keep little kids out of your house as much as possible (they carry more colds).**

- **Put a sign outside your door telling all visitors to immediately wash their hands and slip an oversized T-shirt over their clothes—keep a stack of clean ones by your front door— before they hug you and glom you up with their germs.**

- **Breast-feed if you can.**

- **Immunize your baby, and get your shots, too!**

But if your sweetie does get sick, there are some steps you can take to help her sleep through much of it.

Immunizations: A Blessing to Us All

Hurray! That's the only word to reflect the joy and relief proclaimed by billions of parents through the decades after the discovery of immunizations.

We are incredibly blessed to no longer have tens of thousands of our babies choking from whooping cough, dying from measles and meningitis, or crippled from polio.

To fully protect your baby, make sure he starts his vaccines by two months of age. Why so early? Because some illnesses are especially dangerous during the first months of life.

Whooping cough (also called pertussis) is by far the biggest threat, because it's *super*contagious—any member of your family could accidentally carry it home—and it's found in every single community across America!

Whooping cough slowed dramatically in the 1990s (thanks to active immunization programs). However, in recent years many parents have delayed and skipped their babies' shots.

Bad idea! The number of babies needlessly suffering and dying from this preventable disease has jumped. In 2010–11, California suffered its worst pertussis epidemic in sixty years, with tens of thousands of cases. And antibiotics were rarely helpful.

Influenza is another serious problem that may knock at your door. It causes two hundred thousand hospitalizations and thirty-six thousand deaths annually in the United States. Infants are especially at risk—and even when they only get a mild case, the coughing can ruin sleep for weeks or even months.

I also want to remind *you* to get your shots! Like a caterpillar, you want to wrap your baby in a "cocoon" of protection to keep whooping cough and influenza out of your house. Since newborns can't receive these shots, the key to protecting your baby is to have everyone else in your family immunized. (And make sure your babysitter and nanny are also tested for tuberculosis and hepatitis B.)

Simple Remedies

If your baby gets a cold, try these natural steps to make her more comfortable:

- **NOSE WASHERS.** Put a drop of fresh breast milk in each nostril. (At the end of a feeding, just pick some up from your nipple with an eyedropper.) Sound odd? The immune cells and antibodies in the milk are the only things that fight off a cold! If you're not nursing, you can use a drop of sterile saline (sold at any pharmacy).

- **NOSE SUCKERS.** Babies are nose breathers, so mucus can be a real problem. Buy a nasal bulb syringe (I like the blue ones with the long neck) and ask your nurse or doctor to show you how to use it. Swaddle first (to keep your baby's arms from flailing), put in a drop of breast milk or saline (to loosen the mucus), then suck it all out.

- **NOSE PROTECTORS.** A great nose-protecting tool is a cool mist humidifier. It will keep mucus from hardening in your baby's nose, which is especially important if you live in a dry climate or high altitude. Use distilled water in your humidifier and wash it out every day to keep bacteria from growing in the water.

Oh, and one more thing: ask your doctor about helping your baby breathe easier by elevating the head of her crib just two or three inches. The easiest way to do this is by putting a folded towel under the mattress.

For *Your* Health: Catch All the ZZZZ's You Can!

As artist Ashley Brilliant said, "Sometimes the most urgent and vital thing you can do . . . is take a nap."

Really . . . take a nap! This is a biggie!

Exhaustion is the number one parent complaint after birth. Everyone told you that you'd get worn out during the first few months, but it's always a surprise how bone tired you can get. Especially, *especially* if you're also recovering from a Cesarean section. For some women, the fatigue starts receding after the first month. But for others, it just grinds on month after month.

Furthermore, exhaustion triggers many other serious problems, like marital fights, infections (from colds to mastitis), overeating, car accidents . . . and postpartum depression. (I'll go over some new and important understandings about depression at the end of this chapter.)

So to stay healthy, make sure you get a little relief. Here's how:

- **TAKE NAPS.** This can help make up for your poor nighttime sleep. (Many moms find it easier to nap with the help of white noise and an eye mask to block out the light.)

- **TURN OFF YOUR PHONE.** Put a nice message on your voice mail or answering machine telling people how the baby is doing . . . *and saying that you're not returning calls for the next month.* (That lets you screen calls and ignore all but the most important ones.)

- **SCREEN YOUR VISITORS.** As my mom used to say, "Don't be stupid polite!" A few well-wishers are fine, but only if they're healthy and helpful.

- *EAT WELL.* Have less takeout food (too much salt, sugar, and fat). Ask friends to bring you food that's easy to freeze and reheat (healthy casseroles, veggie lasagna, stews, etc.). And, less time spent shopping, cooking, and cleaning means more time you can sleep.

Stand By Your Man . . . or Your Woman

When we're stressed and exhausted, we tend to take it out on the people around us. That's why a house with a newborn can often seem like Fight Club! So here are some quick reminders for this crazy time.

A Note to Dad

Bend over backward to be nice! Your partner is the mom of your child. She did all the heavy lifting of pregnancy, labor, and delivery. She went through enormous and difficult body changes. She now has to go through all the effort to get back in shape.

The Sleep in America poll found that when someone gets up to help the baby in the middle of the night . . . 89 percent of the time, it's mom. So cut her some slack!

When she complains, let her vent and remember to acknowledge her feelings *before* you ladle out your advice. Don't bug her about cleaning or cooking. Suck it up and help out (even though you're working hard all day—and *you're* tired and stressed, too). Buy her flowers every Friday for two months. This will score *big* points with her friends, and she'll remember your kindness for the rest of her life.

You both may want sleep more than sex. But if you are getting sexually frustrated, please remember that women often have *pelvic exhaustion* after giving birth, and their breasts may be uncomfortably sensitive. Also, be aware that your partner may be embarrassed if her breasts leak during sex or if you're having sex in front of the baby.

But do touch and cuddle. Sex will come.

Postpartum Depression (PPD)

"I waited to become a mother until I was thirty-seven, and I felt totally ready and excited," Loretta said. "That's why I was so disappointed in myself when, a few weeks after my beautiful baby was born, I felt more fear and agitation than excitement. I felt inadequate, like an imposter."

Loretta added, "My body failed me and I needed a Cesarean section. I felt like a blimp. And nursing was really hard because my nipples were flat. It all felt like a catastrophe— like I was watching a bad movie. All I wanted to do was run away . . . from my life, from my husband, and from my sweet— screamy—little baby."

If you've experienced feelings like Loretta's, you're not alone. In fact, studies report that 15 to 40 percent of all new moms develop PPD. That virtually makes PPD a national epidemic! Most have mild "baby blues," but some are very depressed and a few even develop full-blown psychosis.

And there are some aspects of PPD that might surprise you, too:

- **There's no evidence that PPD is caused by hormonal shifts.**
- **PPD can start right after birth or come on months later.**
- **Men can also get PPD. Up to 50 percent of men whose partners get PPD will experience symptoms of depression as well.**

Many, like Loretta, find their depression is not so much a "weepy" shroud as a daily onslaught of panic and worry. Like a black hole, it can rip away a woman's optimism and self-confidence and fill her with feelings of guilt and inadequacy.

Worse yet, exhaustion mixed with a baby's screams may trigger a flood of painful memories (like being yelled at in anger or ridicule). Of course, your baby's cries have no connection to voices creeping in from the past. But PPD can allow forgotten feelings of shame and rage to burst back to the surface.

For decades, experts speculated that the huge hormone shifts of childbirth trigger PPD. But hormonal surges don't explain why depression may start months later or why new dads get PPD, too.

Research suggests that women get nudged (or shoved) into depression by a mix of stresses. These stresses can include anything from being a single parent to family troubles, but three of the most common preventable stress triggers of PPD are exhaustion, persistent infant crying, and having an unsupportive spouse.

The Nuclear Family:
A Dangerous Experiment

All cultures know it's hard being a new mom. That's why many societies reward them with one hundred days of special family care at home, so they can be fed, bathed, and *babied,* too.

But in our society, many parents have lost that communal or family safety net. Even worse, many new parents don't even think they want or need it. They think it's normal for new parents to just *gut it out* on their own.

But nothing could be further from the truth!

The nuclear family—two parents and some kids—is actually a huge experiment, just a century old. And it's one of the most unintelligent and riskiest experiments in human history.

Renowned pediatrician T. Berry Brazelton tells of visiting a small Japanese fishing village where the ancient tradition was to wait on new mothers hand and foot for thirty days. "The new mothers were even fed—bite by bite—and they called their own mothers *Mommy*!" Brazelton recounted that in this community postpartum depression didn't exist.

Of course, few of us live in a village like that—and you can't conjure up nurturing relatives out of thin air. But you *can* call on a neighbor, nanny, or doula to help you out. Getting help is neither an extravagance nor a sign of failure. It's the bare minimum you need . . . and deserve!

So please don't buy into the phony idea that you are supposed to do it all on your own; since the dawn of time few parents ever did.

The PPD/Sleep Link

The connection between fussy, poorly sleeping babies and PPD is a strong one. Researchers at a colic clinic in Rhode Island reported that 45 percent of moms with very irritable young babies had moderate to severe depression. That's a ten times higher incidence of serious PPD than is typical.

Most depressed moms also report that their babies don't sleep well. Interestingly, these moms may not actually sleep fewer hours, but they definitely feel more exhausted. They need an extra hour or two of sleep each day just to stay in balance.

And not only does exhaustion stoke depression; depression increases exhaustion. Moms with PPD often state they can't sleep well because their minds are reeling with concerns and fears. Even when the baby is snoozing, worries keep them awake and spinning thoughts tend to rouse them from light sleep.

Tired moms can totally understand why the ancient Greeks believed that the brothers of the god Sleep (Hypnos)—Blame and Doom (Momus and Moros)—knocked at your door if Hypnos didn't pay you a visit.

Fighting PPD with the 5 S's

After feeling increasingly dejected for a couple of weeks, Rachel reached out for help. She realized that four-week-old Hannah was getting to be too much for her to handle.

She got two part-time helpers to give her a chance to rest, but this made her feel even worse. "The sitters were so calm with Hannah," she said, "I couldn't help but feel that I was bad for her in some way."

I asked Rachel to come to my office. I wanted to teach her the 5 S's to help her get some sleep, but I was also concerned that she was developing PPD. So besides giving her some calming and sleep tips, I encouraged her to make an appointment with a psychologist the following week just in case the 5 S's didn't help.

Fortunately, as soon as Rachel was able to calm Hannah faster and boost her sleep, her depression lifted and her sense of hope began to brighten. The more Hannah slept, the more Rachel began feeling like a good mom.

She told me, "Yesterday, I calmed Hannah in two minutes! I am so relieved! My life has turned around. And I never even had to speak with the psychologist."

Doctors can't do much to solve the money problems, family feuds, or unemployment that can fuel depression, but we can do lots to protect new mothers from the three top PPD triggers: infant crying, sleeplessness, and unsupportive partners.

The 5 S's aren't a miracle cure for PPD, but they can be a real help. Parents who can quickly calm their babies' screams feel more competent and confident. That's why *Happiest Baby* classes have been used in PPD prevention and treatment programs.

At Virtua Health, in New Jersey, for instance, depressed moms taught the 5 S's reported less anxiety and marital stress, more sleep and confidence in their parenting skills, and fewer urges related to harming their babies. And besides turning on the baby's *calming reflex*, white noise can also cover over the chatter in an anxious mother's mind that keeps her awake at night.

One dad wrote, "Sound was the 'secret sauce' for getting our little Selene to sleep. And what was really cool was that the rain track on the white noise CD that helped our baby so much also snookered my depressed, insomniac wife. She stopped waking up with every passing train . . . and started falling asleep in five minutes flat."

The 5 S's can also turn an unsupportive partner into an ally. Time and again, families report that dads who learn baby calming feel great about themselves . . . feel that the baby likes them . . . and are more likely to reach out and offer even more help. This can dramatically lighten the load on a mom's shoulders.

In addition to the 5 S's, there's much more you can do to prevent or reduce PPD. The first step is to talk with your health-care professional, who can check for treatable medical issues that may imitate PPD (like an underactive thyroid) and recommend resources or medication.

Also, try these tips:

- **GET EXERCISE EVERY DAY.** It brightens your spirits, burns off calories, and boosts sleep. Sunlight is a huge help, too. But if it's wintertime or you live in a rainy and gray climate, ask your doctor about prescribing a special SAD light to use one or two hours each morning. (SAD stands for *seasonal affective disorder*, the type of depression people get from long winter nights.)

- **TRY TO EAT BETTER, BUT TAKE A THREE-MONTH VACATION FROM WORRYING ABOUT YOUR WEIGHT.** Getting thinner will happen pretty automatically once you start getting more sleep. Also, there are two supplements that may help fight depression: vitamin D (4000 IU a day) and omega-3 fatty acids (3 grams a day). If you breast-feed, ask your baby's doctor if taking extra vitamin D replaces your infant's need for vitamin drops.

- **REACH OUT.** Find a good friend, a support group, or a hotline so you can share your feelings—*all* of your feelings. And ask your friends to bring a frozen casserole, do some cleaning, or watch the baby so you can take a break.

- **SLEEP EVERY CHANCE YOU GET.** Sleep is like an essential nutrient. So nap when your baby naps . . . doze when your mom comes over . . . sleep whenever you can.

- **TRY A MASSAGE.** *Getting* a massage helps to reduce feelings of depression, and so does *giving* one! Studies show that massaging your baby reduces PPD. So give your baby a little massage every day using a little sweet oil, like sesame or almond. (You can find instructions on giving a perfect baby massage in the book *The Happiest Baby on the Block*.)

Ask for Help Now . . . Pass It Forward Later

Luckily, most parents don't experience PPD. But all new parents—even the happiest, most energetic ones—have one thing in common: they need help!

So don't hesitate to ask for it. Get friends and relatives to pitch in. Hire a nanny or a doula. See if a neighbor can pick up your dry cleaning or fetch some groceries.

Promise me, too, that you won't feel guilty about this for an instant . . . because you're *supposed* to get help and coddling right now. It's good for you, and it's good for your baby.

And here's the deal. Someday, when your child is off in school or all grown up and you have some free time, you can "do for" another new mom or dad who needs help. It's one of those gifts that keeps on giving!

Crib Notes:
Reviewing *The Happiest Baby* Way

- You can *sleep train* your baby's tummy and quickly stretch her sleep! Give your baby frequent feeds during the day and do more efficient nursing (give both sides at each meal) and offer *dream feeds*.

- Prevent night waking by keeping your baby healthy. Simple steps from clean T-shirts to breast milk drops in the nose can help your little sweetie sidestep illnesses and sleep longer.

- Postpartum depression is often triggered by a baby's wails and a mom's exhaustion. You may be able to prevent or lessen your depression by using the *5 S*'s to soothe your baby's cries and boost her nightly sleep.

## CHAPTER FIVE

Q&A: Common Questions About Baby Sleep: Birth to Three Months

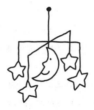

1. When my baby falls asleep after a feeding, should I burp her and risk waking her up?

Yes! You don't want her to spit up her entire meal and need another one. After a feeding, babies get so serene and satisfied that they usually fall back to sleep quickly, especially with the help of white noise and snug swaddling. So it's fine to wake her to do burping or change a diaper.

By the way, it's also a good idea to put ointment on your baby's bottom at night to protect her skin from any pee or poop that might sneak out while she's asleep.

2. I'm confused. Will my baby sleep better if he takes both breasts, or just one to make sure he gets the rich, fatty hindmilk?

Breast milk is fascinating stuff! It changes dramatically during the course of a feeding. The first milk to spurt out (foremilk) is loaded with protein and antibodies, and it has extra water to satisfy your baby's thirst. But after ten to fifteen minutes, as the breast empties, the milk flow slows and gets richer, releasing the creamy, sweet hindmilk.

Some experts worry that feeding a baby for five to ten minutes on each breast will fill the baby with the more watery foremilk and lead to more night waking. They think that the baby must get the rich hindmilk to make him sleepy (like a heavy meal makes us drowsy).

Others believe that babies drink down more milk when they're given both sides during each meal. (More milk flows quickly during the first minutes of a feeding; then it slows down to a slow drip, drip, drip.)

Here is my personal recommendation: try both ways to see what's best for your baby.

If one breast keeps him sleeping four hours at night, there's no need to switch. But if he seems hungry too often or he's gaining weight too slowly, give five minutes on one side and then ten to fifteen minutes (or even longer) on the other. That way, your baby will get the foremilk from both breasts and still get all the hindmilk from the second side. (And any hindmilk left in the breast at the end of a feeding will stay there and just boost the calories of the next meal.)

Interestingly, babies who eat formula sleep fine, despite there being absolutely *zero* difference between the first gulp of milk and the last. So, probably the foremilk/hindmilk issue isn't that important.

3. Why does my baby get up at the crack of dawn?

Even when babies sleep, they still feel, hear, and see. The early morning light filters through their closed eyes, soft spot, and thin skull, turning off their melatonin and turning on their circadian rhythm alarm clock.

You may be able to coax your baby to sleep a little longer by using blackout curtains to shut out the sun's first rays. Also, white noise helps obscure the early morning sounds of birds, dogs, traffic, and the neighbors. And sometimes the sound even helps a baby successfully ignore the early morning light.

4. Is it okay to let my baby sleep on my chest?

I don't recommend it. I once had a couple call me in the middle of the night when their four-week-old baby fell off his father's chest and hit the wall next to the bed. (The dad hadn't intended to sleep like that, but he was so exhausted it happened accidentally.)

Fortunately, that baby wasn't hurt, but a fall like that might have caused a serious injury.

5. Could acid reflux be causing my two-month-old's fussing and frequent waking?

Many, many babies have mild reflux. We just call it *spitting up*. Babies rarely need medicine for this; they just grow out of it over the first four to eight months.

But, in an alarming trend, the number of fussy babies diagnosed with acid reflux has skyrocketed over the past decade. It increased 400 percent just from 2000 to 2003 and has continued to zoom up since then. Yet the best science shows that we are wildly overdiagnosing reflux. Babies should not be treated for acid reflux unless they're failing to gain weight and have over five large vomits per day.

For babies who cry, but are otherwise well, acid reflux medicine is no more helpful than distilled water. Most likely, the abdominal "discomfort" these babies seem to have is just an overreaction to the gastro-colic reflex (the normal waves of peristalsis passing through the digestive system).

In the study of the 5 S's done by the Colorado Department of Public Health, several fussy babies who'd already been placed on acid reflux medication were able to stop taking it after the parents learned how to soothe their crying and promote sleep with the 5 S's.

6. My baby wakes up sweaty, even when the fan is on. Does that mean she's overheated?

Overheating is one thing that can cause sweating. Thirty minutes after your baby falls asleep, check her ears to see if they're red and very warm, and feel her neck to see if it's sweaty.

If she's overheated, swaddle her in a thin muslin blanket with only a diaper on. And use a fan or air conditioner to keep her cool.

But if she's not hot, then her late-night sweating is probably just a sign of her being in deep sleep (stage 3 NREM). In this profound sleep, breathing is slow and the face is totally at peace—but oddly, some of us (babies and grown-ups alike) sweat so much our hair can form wet little ringlets.

7. How can I reverse my one-month-old's day-night confusion?

Here are three easy steps that can usually handle that type of problem in just about a week.

■ **Take lots of daytime walks to get extra sunlight exposure. (Indirect light is best in the summertime, to avoid sunburns.) If it's too cold to go out, get lots of light exposure at home, especially during the early morning, to help set your baby's circadian clock.**

■ **Carry your baby in a sling for long periods of the day (or use a swing) to reinforce the idea that the daytime is an active time.**

■ **Use swaddling and strong, rumbling white noise for all naps and nights.**

## PART II

Sidestepping Infant Sleep Problems: Three to Twelve Months

Chapter 6 looks at the big developmental advances of infancy, and how they can trigger new middle-of-the-night wake-ups. It also busts some more myths (for instance, is Grandma right about cereal and sleep?), explores normal infant sleep patterns, and discusses the best time for your little snoozer to move to his own room.

Chapter 7 shows how to create great sleep cues that don't require mama or dada to be constantly "on call" and how to break bad sleep habits—both your infant's and *yours*. And you'll learn the surprising reason why smart parents start bedtime . . . in the morning! In addition, you'll learn about the worrisome link between poor sleep and childhood obesity.

Chapter 8 explains how to help your infant sleep all night long. You'll learn how to "feed for success" with cluster feeds, calorie shifting, and other tricks—and when to wean swaddling, sound, swinging, and the pacifier. It also clears the air about problems like head banging, teething, and constipation. And finally, I'll share with you the gentlest—and fastest—methods for "sleep training" a baby.

Chapter 9 answers the questions that parents of infants between three and twelve months of age most often ask.

## CHAPTER SIX

"Hello, World!" Your Infant Wakes Up to Life: Three to Twelve Months

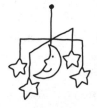

KEY POINTS:

★ Your infant's mind is popping with new interests and challenges! That's fun, but it may also mean less shut-eye for both of you.

★ Now sleep cues start becoming sleep *habits* . . . and they're an excellent way to induce slumber.

★ It's time to toss out five common infant sleep myths, including the big one about cereal and sleep.

★ What's normal sleep for infants? Expect shorter snoozes during the day and longer stretches at night.

★ **Bed-sharing becomes safer and moving your little one to her own room becomes easier . . . your choice!**

Parenting is a stage of life's journey where the milestones come about every fifty feet.

—ROBERT BRAULT

What a Difference a Trimester Makes!

When I ask expectant moms and dads to describe the difference between a newborn and a three-month-old, they usually say, "Hmmm, I don't know . . . one is bigger?" Most don't realize the huge leap their baby will take from being a delicious, fetuslike newborn (who could barely smile) to being a three-month-old nosy little Mr. Social Networker!

But you do. It's only been three months, but I bet your pregnant friends now quiz you like you're a regular baby Wikipedia. You are now an official baby expert!

However, don't rest on your laurels. Depending on what study you read, 15–46 percent of infants suffer from sleep problems sometime during the first year. These can drag on for months, igniting squabbles, exhaustion, overeating, frustration, and hair loss (when you pull it out in frustration!).

So even if your baby is snoozing well now, don't brag about it to your friends. Big changes (weaning swaddling, growth spurts, poop changes) are coming soon that can totally disrupt her slumber (and yours!), and make your little sweetie start waking every three hours—like a newborn—all over again.

And, even if your little friend skates through the next few months, her sleep may get shattered between six and twelve months by a completely new swarm of challenges (teething pain, first colds, adding formula, constipation, new foods, pulling to stand, etc.).

These common disturbers cause so many thorny sleep struggles between three and twelve months that many experts give up and simply tell parents to let their infants "cry it out." But is that really the best we can do? Parents in other cultures think we're crazy to deposit a crying baby in a room—alone—to shout himself into exhaustion.

I'm not saying that crying it out can't work; indeed it can. But it's contrary to one of your biggest parenting goals: building your child's confidence in himself . . . and you.

Fortunately, most infants can be trained to sleep well—and to be more self-sufficient—without leaving them to cry. In the upcoming pages, you'll learn to be an expert in gentle ways to sleep train.

But first . . . let's talk about the exciting advances your little one is going through right now.

Kid's Stuff: What's Going on in Your Child's Mind?

Congrats! Your baby is at the three-month mark . . . and he's now fully "ready to be born." Seriously, look at how big his head and body are now, and you can really appreciate why merciful Mother Nature designed babies to spend the *fourth trimester* on the outside.

Over the next nine months, you'll have tons of fun watching your infant develop into a passionate, curious, self-controlled, and flirtatious member of your family. And even though he's a newcomer to your household, you'll soon have a hard time imagining a world without his smiling face.

But that's not to say he'll *always* be smiling . . . which brings us back to a topic we touched on earlier.

Your Infant's Emerging Temperament

Knowing about your infant's personality is supervaluable because your job is not to raise *a* child . . . it's to raise *your* child.

It's only been a few months, but already you are the world's expert on your child. You're the authority on her sweet smell and funny smile, and on her mood, courage, persistence, and exuberance. Knowing your little one's temperament helps you predict if she'll sleep smoothly during your vacation travels or have trouble with the strange shadows and scents.

Chances are your infant is one of the 40 percent of kids with an easy temperament. These kids are flexible, happy, and not too intense. They love surprises and new situations. They wake up cheerful and ready for the day.

About 25 percent of infants have a challenging temperament—either very sensitive and slow to warm up to people, or spirited and full of beans. These babies will need a little special handling at this stage in life.

Cautious Infants

At five months, when most babies hand out smiles like free samples, cautious infants frown at strangers and glance worriedly at their mom for rescue. These sensitive little munchkins squawk if they're given a new paci, too much light streams in from the hallway, or you try a new perfume.

Cautious infants need regular sleep schedules and routines. So if you have one of these sweet little things, here's my advice: when you get to chapters 7 and 8, make it your mission to use *all* the sleep routines and cues . . . religiously.

Spirited Infants

These little tigers demand lots of attention and hours of movement ("No, Mom, you can't sit down!"). They wait about sixty seconds for their milk to be ready before they erupt in indignation.

Spirited infants are constantly excited by the world. They're the "Me, too!" kids. Since they hate missing even *a moment* of fun, they fight sleep until they're so tired they either conk out mid-giggle or suddenly crumble and turn into total fussbudgets.

For this reason, spirited kids do best when we don't let them get overtired or overexcited before bedtime.

"She's Brilliant!": Infants Are Excellent Students

One of my favorite books on child development, *The Scientist in the Crib*, highlights what little geniuses our young children are.

Now that you're a seasoned parent, you know the *gigantic* advances your child has made. Just a month ago, he could barely keep his eyes from crossing when he looked right at you. Now his eyes can smartly track your movements—even when you're all the way across the room.

As the months pass, your little baby will go from being a blob to being a jock, as his coordination marches down his body. First, he'll gain control of his eyes and face, cooing at will. Next, his neck will strengthen; then he'll be able to suck his fingers without poking his eye. (Watch out, because he'll also start whacking the glasses off your face . . . and grabbing for your hot tea.)

Then will come sitting, crawling, and even standing. (Pulling to stand may create a sleep problem for your nine-month-old if he gets marooned in that position, unable to figure out how to get back down!)

All this movement is endless fun, but it may also make your little friend start fighting against having to *leave the party* when bedtime comes and you have to put him to sleep alone in a flat, boring crib.

Your infant's brain is sprouting a massive amount of new connections or *synapses*. As the neurons develop millions more hookups, her various brain centers can really start working as a team: fast, coordinated, accurate.

Besides the better muscle control I just discussed, you'll witness a big advance in her ability to express feelings (from sadness to fear to joy) and a striking improvement in her *state control*—the ability to stay alert longer, sleep better, and rebound faster from big upsets. (Those waves of colicky crying are quickly becoming a distant memory.)

This improved wiring also leads to better memory. Amazingly, by four to six months, your little one remembers who is family and who is a stranger. (And depending on her temperament, strangers may be seen as fun or a threat.)

Better memory helps explain why your six-month-old goes from great sleep to waking at 2 A.M. ready to play. ("I walked with Mom today. It was fun. Hey, Mom! Wake up, let's walk again!") And it explains why your nine-month-old may protest if you happen to put her down one night without her lovey (or without the *right* lovey!).

And finally, improved memory is also why little *daily routines* become so important in her life. Infants love routines because they create an oasis of predictability in a hectic and uncertain world. A consistent bedtime routine makes your child feel confident and secure. ("Ahh, yes! I know exactly what's about to happen. Kisses, a lullaby . . . and sweet sleep.")

Sleep Cues: Switching from Reflex to Habit

Every day your infant is noticing that some sights and sounds always go together. He's realizing "When I smile, Daddy does, too." In a few months, he'll recognize that "when Mommy points her second finger and looks at something, she wants me to look at it, too" and "when I hear the garage door open, Dad will soon appear."

Between three and five months, the *calming reflex* slowly disappears and the *5 S's* no longer trigger automatic soothing. (Shush an angry ten-month-old and he'll probably shush you right back!) But, this is when *learning* comes to the rescue.

Because of his new ability to make associations, your smart baby is figuring out that his bedtime routine means that play is over . . . it's time for sleep. ("Oh, the white noise, I'll be asleep soon. Oh, I feel tired already!")

White noise and rocking are still calming (even ninety-year-olds are lulled by ocean sounds and rocking chairs), but they only work if your infant is *ready* to be calmed. Now, the *5 S*'s shift from switching on a reflex to becoming reassuring sleep cues, like *teddy bears* of sound and motion.

In the next chapter, I'll discuss how you can use this understanding to create great sleep cues to help you extend your baby's sleep to six, seven, eight hours . . . or more.

Don't Believe It! Common Myths About Sleep at Three to Twelve Months

Besides newborn sleep myths, there are plenty of mistaken ideas about older infants' sleep. Here are five of the most common misconceptions.

MYTH 1: *Infants sleep longer if they're kept awake until they're supertired.*

FACT: Fatigue makes adults sleep better, but it can totally backfire with infants and make them wired and restless.

Earlier, I told you that for newborns, *sleep begets sleep*. This is just as true for older infants. Far from improving sleep, skipping naps and delaying bedtime are the quickest ways to push your baby into screaming meemies and poor sleep.

This is especially the case for infants who are passionately curious. They blink, rub their ears, and fight to stay awake to watch you talking or their big brother clowning around.

Your baby will stay happier, fall asleep faster, and sleep longer when you start his naps and a bedtime routine *before* he's yawning and glassy-eyed.

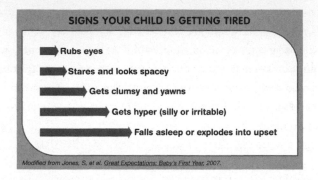

MYTH 2: *Swaddling should be stopped by three months.*

FACT: Parents often hear that babies need their hands free to suck and self-soothe, or that they get dependent on wrapping if it's used too long, or that it interferes with muscle development.

Actually, babies do best with swaddling for four months, or longer.

Babies have tons of time to practice finger sucking when they're unswaddled during the day. Infants don't get dependent on the swaddling. And finally, babies have plenty of time to work on rolling and sitting during their hours of unwrapped play during the day.

I recommend swaddling for at least four months. That's because swaddling makes it harder for babies to roll to the stomach, the risky position for SIDS. And some jittery, uncoordinated little kids benefit from wrapping until five, six, or seven months, when they're finally mature enough to stop accidentally whacking themselves in the face. (I'll discuss weaning swaddling on page 179.)

MYTH 3: *You should be able to train your four-month-old to sleep through the night.*

FACT: Well, I guess that depends on how you define *sleep through the night*.

After birth, your baby will need frequent feedings to fuel the rapid growth of his body and brain. (Your baby's body *doubles* in size during the first six months. Imagine how many times a day you'd need to eat to do that!)

By three or four months, most babies' brains are mature enough to sleep for at least a six-hour stretch without needing to be fed. But if you insist that sleeping through the night means snoozing from 10 P.M. to 6 A.M., you'll need all the routines I describe in the next two chapters. Without that help, up to 30 percent of infants still can't sleep eight hours straight by their first birthday.

MYTH 4: *Giving rice cereal in the evening boosts a baby's sleep.*

FACT: For decades, grandmas—and doctors—taught that feeding babies a spoon or two of cereal would fill their stomach and keep them sleeping all night. But several studies show that bedtime cereal does *nothing* to promote sleep.

Of course, when you think about it for a minute, you realize it is a totally crazy idea to begin with. Baby rice cereal is *much* less filling (and *much* less nutritious) than rich breast milk or formula. Milk is a mix of fats, carbohydrates, and proteins that turns into pellets of protein curd in the stomach and is slowly digested. Milk also has lots of other satisfying nutrients, like sleep-inducing tryptophan.

Cereal, on the other hand, is just white starch (and a touch of iron).

So the idea that a tablespoon of quick-digesting starch could improve on the job done by eight ounces of warm, rich milk is nuts. (And rice is a silly first food anyway, with almost no redeeming nutritional benefit.)

MYTH 5: *Babies need solid food at six months for good sleep.*

FACT: Okay, feeding is fun! But there's absolutely no rush.

Babies love watching us eat, and most six-month-olds are grabbing at our forks. (But they grab at anything we're holding!) And let's be honest: most of us are just dying to spoon some food into those gorgeous, drooly little mouths.

But it's wrong to think that solid food is becoming important at this age. In fact, milk is still the nutritional powerhouse for your six-month-old. It is rich, complex, and fattening. Baby food, on the other hand, is what supermodels eat when they're on super strict diets—carrots, apples, and peas.

At six months, milk makes up 95 percent of your baby's calories (and food is more entertainment than nutrition). By nine months, milk still makes up about 75 percent of the calories, and by one year, it's a good 50 percent of your child's diet.

So make sure your baby isn't skipping milk during the day to fill up on food. Otherwise, she's going to start popping awake hungry all night long.

Sleep: What's Normal at This Stage?

As your child's development takes a giant step forward, a more regular sleep pattern begins to take shape. The sleep statistics below, provided by Sleepedia and based on a national sample, show you how this will change as he grows and develops.

By three months, your baby's shreds of sleep are increasingly woven into longer naps and nights. He's getting better at being soothed back to sleep (by himself or you) and not erupting into tears.

Yet some aspects of your infant's slumber are similar to those in the first months. For example, both newborns and three-month-olds nap a lot and sleep about fourteen out of twenty-four hours each day.

The National Sleep Foundation's 2004 Sleep in America poll of fifteen hundred families discovered that most infants nap three to four hours during the day, fall asleep within ten minutes of lights-out and sleep ten hours at night, with 71 percent waking at least once a night (and slightly less than half waking two or more times).

Of course, these are averages, and there's a big variation from one child to the next. About 5 percent of infants sleep as little as ten hours per twenty-four hours, and 5 percent sleep a whopping eighteen hours!

And, as the year passes, you can expect to see:

- **MORE NIGHT SLEEP.** Night sleep jumps from eight hours at birth to nine hours at three months, to eleven hours at one year.

- **LONGER STRETCHES OF NIGHT SLEEP.** Half of babies can sleep five hours (from midnight to 5 A.M.) by two months—and half can sleep eight hours straight (from 10 P.M. to 6 A.M.) by five months. (And they can do even better when we use good sleep cues, like white noise.)

- **GRADUALLY LESS DAYTIME SLEEP.** Daytime sleep shrinks from eight hours at birth, to four and a half hours at three months to about three hours at one year.

Melatonin: Nature's Built-In Elixir of Sleep

"You're killing my melatonin!" That's the gentle reminder my wife gives me if I accidentally turn the light on while she's sleeping.

Around four months of age, your baby's sense of day and night (circadian rhythm) is getting much better, thanks to the fantastic dance of neural messengers in his brain. Now, every night brings a surge of *melatonin*.

As you'll recall, melatonin is the body's natural sleep hormone, released from the pineal gland deep within the brain. Bright light shuts melatonin off, helping us to stay alert and active in the day, and darkness triggers its release to ease us back into sleep.

This blessed substance is why your infant now sleeps less in the day and more at night. And it's why I strongly recommend you dim your house lights thirty to sixty minutes *before* bedtime and keep bright lights away from your little guy's room after you put him down for the night.

Where's Your Infant Sleeping Now?

By four months, your babe will probably outgrow the coziness of her bassinet. And you have two big decisions about where your baby will sleep next:

1. In a crib . . . or your bed?
2. In your room . . . or in hers?

Let's look at your choices.

Crib or Bed-Sharing?

Moving your young infant to a crib from a bassinet or cosleeper is pretty easy. A couple of weeks before you make the switch, just start a routine of some fun, quiet play together in the crib each day (a little massage is perfect). For infants over six months, it also helps to place a small, silky blanket or cuddly teddy bear in the crib as a lovey (transitional object). And of course, continuing your white noise will create a reassuringly familiar bridge to smooth the transition.

On the other hand, you may decide to bring your darling into your bed. The coziness of having your little one in bed with you is hard to resist!

Earlier, I mentioned SIDS increases in *newborns* who bed-share. However, studies show that after four months (or, for premature babies, four months past the due date), you can bed-share safely as long as you still *make every effort to avoid bed-sharing dangers* (see page 48).

Yet bed-sharing can still backfire on you. Many studies show that bed-sharing babies wake more frequently at night. The Sleep in America poll found that 23 percent of bed-sharing parents reported sleep problems, versus 13 percent of non-bed-sharers.

Another study found that while many families loved bed-sharing, 30 to 40 percent felt it was a problem for their child and family. They got into the habit only because they didn't know how else to settle their infant. And the same study found that parents who bed-shared were three times more likely to say they had significant stress in their marriage.

So feel free to make the decision that is right for your family, but please do it safely.

Wiggly Worms: Don't Let Your Infant Fall Off the Bed

Five-month-old Martin and his parents were on a long-awaited vacation. Maja and Dimitri had rented a room in a rustic old inn. It was high on a hill with views over the town, high ceilings, and beautiful stone floors.

As they unpacked their bags, they placed Martin in the middle of the huge bed and turned their backs for a few seconds. Suddenly, there was a thud and a scream. Martin had rolled off the bed and fallen—headfirst—onto the stone pavers.

Feeling terrified and guilty, they spent all night in an ER with their baby, having to rely on unknown doctors, getting blood tests and brain scans. He suffered a huge blood blister under his skin, but fortunately there was no fracture or bleeding inside the brain.

Never leave your baby unattended on an adult bed . . . even
if she is just two weeks old . . . even if she has never rolled
before . . . even if you will only be away for a second! I have
seen many, many young babies who fell off their parents' beds.
Not all were as lucky as Martin.

Moving Out: Going from Your Room to the Nursery

At three months, 85 percent of babies are still in their parents'
room. Room sharing is superconvenient, so there's no rush to
move your baby out.

Feeding is easy when your tyke is in a bassinet or cosleeper
next to your bed. There's no middle-of-the-night hike down a
cold, dark hall, and no struggling to fall back asleep again. And
you get to hear your baby's white noise, which can help *you* sleep
better, too.

Also, room sharing is safer. You can hear if your infant is
having a problem, and just being near her reduces her risk of SIDS.

Yet, by the first birthday about 70 percent of parents have
moved their baby to another room.

When's the best time for this move? I recommend doing it by
six to seven months. After that, infants become much more tuned
in to the particulars of their surroundings and may have trouble
with the change.

Also, by eight months, many babies suddenly notice—and really
care—if there's no one nearby. This can especially be a problem if
they're used to having company in their room, but now find themselves left totally alone. Separation worry is especially stressful
for babies with a sensitive or cautious temperament.

When you make the move, don't be shocked if your little one
protests for a few nights when you leave. If this happens, I recommend you pick her up right away and comfort her (don't talk too
much or nurse her; otherwise you will accidentally be encouraging her protests). As she calms, put your little love down again.

If she fusses again, pick her up. Repeat this routine as often as needed. As long as you pick her up as soon as she fusses (and use white noise), it rarely goes on more than thirty minutes.

Here are some additional ways to ease your baby into the change:

- Spend more time in her room one to two months *before* making the switch. Use her room for pleasant, quiet times like feedings, massages, singing, naps, or rocking.

- During the transition, continue all the great routines and sleep cues she loves, like the bedtime routine, white noise CD, lovey, and pacifier.

Regardless of Where Your Baby Beds . . . How Well Are You Sleeping?

After calming Ella and placing her down for a nap, Carol herself was so tired she leaned hard against the wall. Only it wasn't the wall . . . it was the open window of her second-story apartment! Carol knocked out the screen, but she was able to grab onto the window frame to keep herself from falling.

Watching your baby blossom during infancy is one of the greatest gifts you'll receive in life. Each flirty smile and happy chuckle you witness is a treasure.

But to enjoy these delicious moments, you'll need to be *awake* for them. If you're like Carol, you're still sleepwalking through much of your baby's infancy . . . and that means you're missing out on a lot of the fun. It also means that, like Carol, you might be putting yourself or your baby at risk.

Fortunately, help is on the way! In the next two chapters, you'll learn how to get your curious infant to sleep, keep her asleep, and extend her slumber by an hour or two . . . and all with few or no tears.

- Between three and five months, the *calming reflex* slowly disappears.

- Even as the *calming reflex* fades, the *5 S's* continue to be *excellent sleep cues*. They automatically get your baby in the mood to sleep.

- For a much easier bedtime, dim your house lights thirty to sixty minutes *before* bedtime and keep bright lights away from your baby after you put her down for the night.

- White noise is a big help when you want to move your baby out of your bedroom into her own.

## CHAPTER SEVEN

Helping Your Infant Get to Sleep: Three to Twelve Months

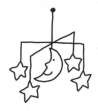

KEY POINTS:

★ Keeping a sleep diary can help you figure out why your infant isn't snoozing well.

★ Why does your little one have trouble sleeping? Overexcitement? A disturbance like teething or outside noise? You need better sleep cues? You picked the wrong bedtime?

★ The biggest habits that lead to poor sleep are bed-sharing, falling asleep while being held or fed, and being put in bed asleep.

- ★ Good sleep can help protect your infant—and you—against obesity.
- ★ Routine is your friend. And surprisingly, the best time to start your bedtime routine is in the *morning*!
- ★ The *5 S*'s are still a key to good sleep. And now other great sleep cues—from loveys to lavender—can help, too.

There was never a child so lovely but his mother was glad to get him to sleep.

—Ralph Waldo Emerson

The Wonderful World of Routines

To grown-ups, the word *routine* sounds a little dull. We get bored doing the same thing, day in and day out. But your little one doesn't feel that way at all. Infants love routines! And as you'll soon see, making your child's bedtime routine as predictable as sunset will be your best tool for boosting her sleep . . . and getting hours of extra rest for yourself.

Little routines fill your infant with the feeling of being smart and loved. And her happiness—and better behavior—will make you feel like a great parent, too!

Researchers have found that 75 percent of parents who say nighttime is easy use a regular, predictable bedtime routine at least five nights a week.

In a study of 405 children (seven to thirty-six months old), sleep expert Dr. Jody Mindell asked parents to use a simple three-step routine (bath, massage, and quiet cuddling or singing a lullaby). Parents put their kids in bed thirty minutes after the end of the bath.

Within two weeks, the children fell asleep faster and had fewer and shorter night awakenings. Among children seven to eighteen months old, continuous sleep increased from almost seven hours to eight and a half. And as a bonus, the routine also reduced moms' tension, anger, fatigue, and confusion.

But good bedtime routines don't just happen. They take planning—and here's one of the biggest surprises to most new parents: the bedtime routine actually starts *early in the day.*

The Happiest Baby Way

THINK AHEAD!—BEDTIME STARTS IN THE MORNING

What you do with your infant during the day makes a big difference in how things go at night. So set yourself up for nighttime success by starting when the sun comes up! Here's how:

- **GET OUTDOORS.** Get your babe outside for a daily dose of sunlight (especially before noon).

- **GET SOUND AND MOTION.** Rhythms throughout the day set a calming tone. Long walks, swings, and slings are great during the day, and swaddling and white noise during naps.

- **STAY ON SCHEDULE.** Create a flexible schedule to keep your infant from getting overtired during the day and to keep her on track for your bedtime target (more about this later).

- **AVOID STIMULANTS.** If you're breast-feeding, avoid "uppers" like dark chocolate and coffee (see page 14).

- **ENCOURAGE POOPING.** Some nice belly massage and knee-to-tummy exercises will help your little one to poop during the day, so nighttime sleep isn't disturbed by grunting. (Speak to your doctor if your infant is having firm or hard stools.)

Prebed Calming Pleasures

Our homes are busy at night, filled with bright light, noise, and lots of activity. All this can overexcite nosy little infants. No wonder they put up a fuss when they're suddenly put in a dark, quiet, still room . . . all alone! To help your infant begin winding down for the night, I recommend you get her "in the mood" with a few simple steps you can do thirty to sixty minutes before the sleep routine starts:

- Dim the lights in your house (reduce them 75 percent, about as bright as candlelight).

- Turn off noisy TVs, video games, music, and so on.

- Switch off your phone.

- Turn on some white noise (as loud as a soft shower).

- Enjoy some quiet play together (like a massage or warm bath) . . . not roughhousing. (One tip: If your little scuba friend gets *more* revved with a bath, you may want to save it for the morning.)

Infant Massage—the Magic of Touch

Touch is our oldest, deepest, most emotional sense. And for babies, it's a profound experience. Amazingly, cuddling is as important for healthy development of a baby's body and brain as milk.

In fact, in some ways touch is even more beneficial than milk. While stuffing your baby with an excess of milk won't make her any healthier, the more loving caresses you give her, the stronger and happier she'll be. Research out of Israel has shown that touch even helps to adjust your baby's melatonin levels and gets her day/night cycle better regulated.

And, as an extra bonus, giving your baby a massage also lowers *your* stress, anxiety, and depression and boosts your self-esteem.

The goal of massage is to help your infant calm and prepare for sleep. So warm the room, turn down the lights, cover her body with a soft towel to avoid chills, and rub a little slippery stuff (like cocoa butter or almond, avocado, or coconut oil) between your hands. Play your white noise quietly in the background *plus* a lullaby or other relaxing music. And enjoy! (You can find detailed instructions on giving a great baby massage in the book *The Happiest Baby on the Block*.)

Best Bedtime Habits: The *5 S*'s, Loveys, and More

The most successful parents know that by the time the *official* bedtime routine starts, their child should already be cleaned, changed, and halfway to winding down for the night.

Now, let's look at the sleep cues you'll layer on during the last twenty to thirty minutes of your bedtime routine to help your little one sweetly float into sleep: the 5 S's, warm milk, storytime, loveys, and *wake-and-sleep*.

The 5 S's

Although the *calming reflex* is fading away, the 5 S's continue to be delicious sleep cues, helping your infant feel cozy and serene. (White noise and swaddling relax your infant's muscles and calm her heartbeat.)

In the newborn chapters, I described each S in detail. Here's a quick look at how to use them with your infant's bedtime routine as she gets older.

SWADDLING

Rachel and Jeff's twins, Ari and Grace, slept swaddled until six months. But the record in my practice goes to Kerry and Robert's daughter, Molly Ann . . . the baby who didn't want to grow up. She loved being bundled until the ripe old age of ten months.

I recommend that you use swaddling for at least four months. However, many babies need it for five, six, or seven months . . . or, like Molly Ann, even longer. (See page 179 for directions on weaning swaddling.) And, *a note of warning:* many infants start waking during the night as soon as the swaddle is removed . . . *unless their parents continue using white noise!*

And, as mentioned earlier, you can continue swaddling your child even after she has begun rolling over as long as you secure her into a *fully reclined* swing or a *fully reclined* infant seat (as described on page 78).

SIDE/STOMACH POSITION

The side and stomach positions are still comforting ways of holding your infant as she nods off to sleep. But when you place your baby down, it should only be on her back.

By four months, about 80 percent of the SIDS risk has passed. That's a very good thing because your baby is now capable of flipping herself from the back to the stomach, so you really no longer have control over her position. Only after your little bug is out of the swaddle (usually around four or five months) will it be safe for her to sleep tummy down. But, just to be on the safe side, I recommend you continue placing her to sleep on the back for the first year.

Of course, to avoid problems you should continue to follow the rules of safe sleeping (see page 53) and do the daily tummy time exercises (see page 55).

SOUND

*Karly, the mother of nine-month-old Matilda, found her own
special lullaby to soothe her baby to sleep—"We Will Rock
You," by Queen.*

*"Regular lullabies had no effect on our high-energy baby,"
she told me. "But one day we discovered that the Queen song
immediately stopped her crying, and the heavy beat got her to
fall into deep sleep in under a minute! From then on, just one
or two repeats of the song would always put her to sleep."*

Sound is as important for good sleep as swaddling! In fact,
once swaddling is weaned, white noise becomes the key sleep cue.

Even if your baby is sleeping well without it, I strongly advise
you to use rumbly white noise for all naps and night—about as
loud as a shower—to help her sleep even better and to prevent the
sleep struggles that so often are suddenly triggered by teething,
growth spurts, and so on.

As the months pass, your infant is getting more and more interested in the world. And that nosiness means that she's much more
likely to pop awake from any little distraction (outside sounds,
bright light from the hallway, teething discomfort, a little gas,
etc.). And if her room is totally quiet, she'll fill that silence with
a yell for you to come cuddle her . . . or to play. These middle-of-
the-night wakings are especially common after you take away the
comforting snuggle of the swaddling blanket.

However, if you're playing familiar white noise sounds, your
little princess may not even notice the disturbance. And even if
she is awakened, she's much more likely to dive right back into
sleep if she is surrounded by the reassuring rumble of white
noise. (If your baby is new to white noise, see the tips on page 72.)

Note: Many infants become so curious at this age that they
require a rougher sound (like a hair dryer or vacuum sound played
as loud as a regular shower) to obscure outside disturbances and
bring them back into sleep.

Now is also the time that you may want to play another type of sound, *in addition to her white noise*: lullabies. Bedtime lullabies add another cue that your baby will learn to recognize as a signal welcoming her back to sweet slumber.

While Queen was just the ticket for Matilda, most babies (and parents) prefer soft singing or gentle lullaby music. In fact, the word *lullaby* means "to sing to sleep," so the tempo is slow and rhythmic—usually one beat per second, just like your heart. The best lullabies have a smooth, regular pace with no sudden changes or loud parts.

But . . . music can actually wake infants up when it's used all night long.

So for great sleep, use white noise *at the same time* as the music. Play the sound softly in the background and the music a little louder during your routine, then turn the white noise back up to shower intensity and allow it to continue after the music ends . . . and straight through until morning.

SWINGS

All babies love being rocked before bed, but only about 5 to 15 percent of infants need the fast motion of a swing all night to help them sleep.

If you plan on using the swing for your infant's sleep, it's important that you ask your doctor's permission and make sure you're using the swing safely and correctly (see page 78 for these safety rules).

SUCKING

The last of the 5 S sleep cues is sucking. Nursing your baby is profoundly calming, and so is a bottle of warm formula. And a bedtime pacifier not only helps satisfy your baby's sucking urge, but it also may reduce SIDS.

Some parents worry that pacifier or thumb sucking is a sign of anxiety or that it will last forever. Actually, this sucking is a very effective way to self-soothe. And most kids give up pacis and finger sucking after one to two years, so you don't have to worry that your child will go to college with a binky dangling from her lips.

One caution about using sucking as a sleep cue is to always pair it with the *wake-and-sleep* technique (see page 88). In other words, if your sweetie has fallen asleep in your arms while sucking, make sure you wake her a tiny bit when you lower her into the crib for the night.

And here's another caution: Many parents let their infants have a bottle in bed. That can be a real problem, because milk and fruit juice contain a lot of sugar (juice has as much sugar as soda!). So long feedings can actually lead to cavities once the teeth start appearing (more on this in chapter 8). If you offer a bottle at bedtime—or nurse your baby in bed with you—don't let her suck for more than thirty minutes. If she still wants more, consider giving her a bottle of pure herbal tea, like mint or chamomile.

Also, if your infant is getting frequent ear infections, ask your doctor if they might be triggered by drinking from a bottle or sucking on a pacifier in bed.

Another *S*: Smell

Lavender is a beautiful purple flower, and the essential oil from this flower has been used for centuries as an aromatherapy treatment to promote calmness, relaxation, and sleep. One ancient remedy for poor sleep was to place a small pillow filled with lavender flowers in your bed.

Only a few small medical studies have been done to scientifically evaluate lavender's calming and sleep-inducing benefits, but the results have generally been positive. Even if the evidence isn't yet strong, I like using it because many infants are very keyed in to smells. They recoil from bad odors and love the scent of their mom's hair and delicious food. So a lovely smell from the crib can become a welcome cue that a wonderful bedtime routine and sweet sleep are about to arrive.

If that sounds like fun to you, try rubbing a few drops of essential lavender oil on the posts of the crib and the sides of the mattress (places where your baby can smell it but can't lick it off). I bet you'll love the smell, too! Lavender oil should never be taken orally, so keep it out of your child's reach.

Once you have your S's in place, here are additional cues that will make your little one's nighty-night routine even more comforting.

Reading

This is a sleep cue with a big bonus! In addition to relaxing your little cherub, reading is the gateway to learning and to your child's ultimate success in school and at work. So it's a wonderful habit to start building early.

Of course, your five-month-old doesn't understand the words you say. But she'll *love* hearing your animated voice, and she'll show more and more interest in looking at the things that you also show interest in.

Many parents find that reading is one of the most enjoyable parts of the bedtime routine.

Loveys: Your Little One's First Friend (Besides You!)

Another great sleep cue is giving your sweetie a cozy, cuddly *lovey* to help him fall asleep.

We all remember Linus in the *Peanuts* cartoon dragging his beloved blankie behind him. And Calvin had Hobbes the tiger, and Christopher Robin loved Winnie-the-Pooh. Did you have a lovey when you were growing up? A blankie or teddy? If you or your partner carried around a Raggedy Ann until she was raggedy, your child will probably like one, too. That's because falling in love with these cuddlies is a strong genetic trait.

Kids love loveys! I've seen them cling to diapers, silk scarves, and all sorts of toys. For years, my little patient Alex was "hooked" on sleeping with his Captain Hook's hook.

Yet, only a third of families employ sleep cues like white noise or loveys. I think that may be because many parents have been frightened by experts who caution that using loveys creates an unhealthy dependency. So wrong!

Parents who turn their backs on loveys are missing a *huge* opportunity! These cuddly friends actually help infants build confidence and security. And they're available anytime—day or night. So a lovey is a very, very *good* habit—and it's especially comforting during times of stress (like an illness or a parent's absence) and for babies with cautious, sensitive temperaments.

From three to six months, the only safe lovey is a pacifier and white noise (which is like an "auditory lovey"). After six months, you can introduce a handkerchief-sized silky blanket or hand-sized cuddly stuffed animal.

But make sure you always have a backup! Losing a lovey is traumatic for a child. Every couple of weeks, rotate your baby's two loveys. That allows you to keep them clean and to have them both develop the same comforting feel and smell.

And also make sure your baby's lovey doesn't have any little pieces (like button eyes or beads in the stuffing) that can be a choking risk or get stuck up the nose.

"Wake-and-Sleep"—the Cherry on Top of Your Bedtime Routine

The last part of your baby's bedtime routine is allowing him to fall asleep on his own. I talked about doing this with your newborn, but it's very important at this stage as well.

If your little guy falls asleep before you place him in the crib, wake him a tiny bit after you put him down. You can do this by changing his diaper, tickling him, or putting your cool hand on his head. He should open his eyes for several seconds, or at least moan and push your hand away a couple of times, and then settle himself back into sleep.

I know this goes against every parental instinct! But it is *the key step* in your little one's education on how to soothe himself back to sleep when he wakes at night. And with the help of the *5 S*'s, a tummy full of milk, and a lovey, he should be able to quickly fall back to sleep.

However, if your little buddy does squawk when you rouse him, just do a tom-tom pat on his back or jiggle the crib quickly until he settles back down. If that doesn't work, pick him up, soothe him, and put him down again. (Jostle him to wake him again if he's fallen asleep before you lay him back down.)

Still Having Problems? It's Time to Take Action

Are you still struggling with sleep problems? Do you pray each night for your tyke to "grow out of it" soon?

Well, I know you don't want to hear this . . . but kids usually don't just outgrow their sleep struggles. These troubles typically persist until you do something to bring them under control. So if you've been waiting patiently and your child's sleep still isn't shaping up—even though you're doing all of the 5 S's and following a great sleep routine—it's time to make a new plan.

The First Step to Success: Figure Out Where You Are Now

The first thing to determine before you plan your sleep strategy is: Does your baby *really* have a sleep problem?

If your baby sleeps eight hours a night (say, from 9 P.M. to 5 A.M.) and naps three hours a day, that may be as good as it gets. Not every baby is going to sleep ten hours straight, or fall asleep and wake up exactly when you want.

But odds are, if you think your little one has a sleep problem, you're right. So your next step is to gather some clues.

In general, I'm not a big one for lists and diaries. If a feeding happens an hour early or a nap an hour late that day, no big deal. But unless you keep notes, it's hard to remember how long your infant slept, how often he awakened, and what it took to help him back to sleep.

A daily diary (see appendix) also allows you to share your concerns with your doctor and will help you keep track of your progress as you work to resolve the problem.

So before monkeying around with bedtime changes, take a few days to notice if your little one is overtired before you put him down (wired and irritable or yawning and bleary-eyed) or wide-awake (happy and playful).

Jot down the times you see early signs of fatigue. Also, take a week to carefully record your infant's key sleep events:

- **Naps (time and duration)**
- **Length of bedtime routine (including the details of the routine)**
- **Time and duration of night awakenings (also list your response)**
- **Time of morning waking**

And, while you're at it, mark down the other big events of the day, like meals, crying jags, and poops.

I've included a *wake/sleep diary* at the back of the book. These diaries are also supercute souvenirs, so hang on to it when you're done with your data collecting. You'll love sharing this with your child many years from now, when he's married with kids of his own!

Pinpointing What's Causing the Problem

Your diary should help you see why your baby is having trouble nodding off. The four top reasons to consider are overexcitement before bedtime, something is bugging her, you're using the wrong bedtime cues, or you picked the wrong bedtime.

Your Infant Is Overexcited

Sometimes parents accidentally teach their babies to expect high excitement at night. This is especially common when parents are away at work all day and return home wanting to *play*.

Out of love (or guilt), you may accidentally overstimulate your infant with roughhousing right before bedtime. But as you might imagine, it's hard for your little bird to switch in just minutes from giggly fun—with the lights as bright as the noontime sun—to being alone in dark silence. (Hmmm, can you do that?) So be sure to dim the lights and stop the tickling well before lights-out.

Overexcitement can also result from giving your little one a stimulant (like caffeine, chocolate, herbal supplements, or decongestants), either directly or through your breast milk.

Something's Bugging Your Baby

Your infant may have trouble falling asleep because something's bothering her. It may be outside her body (like noise, bright lights, bad smells, or a room that's too hot, cold, or stuffy) or inside (like hunger, a stuffy nose, gas, or sore gums).

If your baby's nursery is chilly, put socks on her feet and warm the sheets a little with a hot water bottle for five to ten minutes before popping her in the crib.

But don't put a hat on her! Hats can get pushed down and cover the face as babies wiggle around. And since newborns lose 25 percent of their body heat through their heads, a hat may also cause overheating. If you're not sure what to do, ask your doctor.

Is Emotional Stress Upsetting Your Infant?

Infants can get stressed just like grown-ups. If your child resists sleep, take a minute to make sure her problem isn't a sign of stress. She may be troubled by:

- Yelling or fighting—in real life or on TV

- Scary situations, including barking dogs, loud noises, an unfamiliar bedroom, or new or unfriendly people (a new sitter or teacher, or even a grandma who hasn't visited in a while)

- Separations, such as having to stay with sitters or having a regular caregiver suddenly leave

These can especially upset fragile, supercautious infants who tend to get scared, lonely, and extracranky when unexpected changes occur.

If you think stress is part of the problem, do what you can to protect your honey from these upsets and start a great bedtime routine to get her back in balance.

Your Infant Learned the Wrong Habits

This is probably the number one cause of infant sleep problems in America!

We teach our infants habits that make them dependent on us

rather than ones that build confidence and self-calming ability. The most common habits that lead to poor sleep are bed-sharing and being put in bed asleep.

For example, the Sleep in America poll found that:

- **Sixty percent of infants are usually rocked to sleep (which is wonderful for newborns but can become a problem later on).**

- **Seventy-five percent of infants fall asleep every night nursing or drinking a bottle.**

- **Many infants bed-share, which makes it easy for them to insist that their parents soothe them back to sleep—each time they awaken.**

- **As previously mentioned, only a third of parents use *independence-building* sleep cues like white noise or loveys every night.**

Doctors in Rhode Island found that three- and eight-month-old infants fell asleep *easily*—at bedtime and after nighttime awakenings—if they used loveys and pacifiers. The doctors also reported that all the poorly sleeping eight-month-olds—about one in three infants—were put into their cribs already *asleep* . . . and *none* routinely received a lovey!

Being your baby's sleep aid is fun and cuddly, and I'm all in favor of it as long as *you're* happy with it (and you take precautions like bed-sharing safely). But if you're tired and frustrated, this is the right moment to help your infant learn some new habits. Here are clues that it's time for a change:

- **YOU'RE EXHAUSTED: You're overeating; short-tempered with your toddler or husband; spacing out at work; driving dangerously because you're so tired; feeling depressed; or considering smoking cigarettes again.**

- **YOU'RE FRUSTRATED: You don't know what to do about your infant's sleep resistance, night waking, dependence** on bed-sharing, and frequent night nursing. And you are bickering a lot with your spouse.

- **YOUR CHILD'S UNHAPPY:** She's extracranky; cries at everything; has no patience; seems overtired; gets superirritable at bedtime; or wakes crying during the night.

If you're seeing these trouble signs, it's time to swap your problematic sleep cues for ones that boost sleep *and* nurture your tot's calm, confidence, and competence. Don't get me wrong . . . you should give your little lovebug *tons* of holding, rocking, patting, and suckling. But to avoid sleep problems *later,* you need to focus on sleep cues and routines *now* that will teach her to self-soothe.

The best way to start removing a dependence on being held and rocked to doze off is to use the *wake-and-sleep* technique every time you put your little one down to sleep.

Can Poor Sleep Make Your Infant Obese?

There's lots of evidence that poor sleep causes weight problems for adults (see page 224) and kids. And two recent studies hint that the same is true during infancy.

In the first study, Penn State researchers found that breatfed babies whose parents used the 5 S's (along with some other general parenting tips) slept longer. And the better-sleeping kids had less obesity at one year of age if the moms also followed a simple dietary plan (not to give foods before six months and to comfort fussing with a cuddle before giving a feed).

In the second study, a Harvard team found a 100 percent higher risk of being overweight among three-year-olds who slept less than twelve hours a day during infancy (at six, twelve, and

Your Bedtime Timing Is Off

Infants fight bedtime if they're confused by an irregular or inconsistent bedtime (for instance, when you travel across time zones
or switch to daylight savings) or if bedtime is too early or late.

Most infants fall asleep easily and sleep longer when they're
put down *before* they get tired and bug-eyed. The Sleep in America
poll found that overtired children take almost 20 percent longer
to fall asleep! In other words, *being overtired makes kids wired.* (This
is particularly true for superspirited infants who get increasingly
rebellious.)

The average three-month-old's bedtime is around 9:30 P.M.
Yet, as infants get older their bedtime gets *earlier*, dropping to
8:30 P.M. . . . and earlier. Researchers in Pittsburgh found that
infants who went to bed before 9 P.M. slept significantly longer
overall (13 hours) than infants who went down after 9 P.M. (11.8
hours). But if you push for a bedtime that's too early, your little
buddy may not be tired.

Is bedtime *too early?* Look for these clues:

- Your infant fights falling asleep for thirty to sixty minutes.
- She shows no sign of fatigue at bedtime.
- She wakes up in the middle of the night or very early the next day, refreshed and ready to go.

Is bedtime *too late?* Look for these clues:

- Your munchkin fights falling asleep for thirty to sixty minutes.

- **She's irritable and moody and falls asleep during the day in the car or stroller and takes naps that are over two hours long.**

- **She's clearly overtired at bedtime (rubbing her eyes, blinking, yawning, cranky).**

If you think bedtime is too early, try pushing your routine *fifteen minutes later* every two to three nights.

If you think bedtime is too late, try starting your routine *fifteen minutes earlier* every two to three nights. Either approach should work within a week or two.

Sleep Schedules: Solving Problems with Loving Consistency

I'm not a fan of scheduling your infant's life down to the minute. But having a *flexible* routine can be a real help if:

- **Your baby's not sleeping well: She's a sensitive, persnickety child who falls apart if her nap is too late; gets cranky when she's overtired; resists sleep; wakes too often; or wakes too early in the morning.**

- **You need order in your day: You're juggling lots of responsibilities—other kids, a job, a household—and you need to be extraefficient.**

Here's a simple approach to scheduling that can help you ease your little tyke into a better feeding and sleep routine and get your day organized.

1. FIRST, FIND OUT EXACTLY WHAT'S GOING ON

If you're like most parents, one day blurs into the next. So before you start shifting your infant's schedule, keep a daily wake/sleep diary for several days. As I've mentioned, this will help you quickly identify your infant's typical pattern. (See page 339 for a sample diary.)

2. NEXT, SET GOALS

After the first months, a good goal is to put your little one down to nap about every two to three hours during the day. Keep naps to under two hours. (By the first birthday, her naps will occur every three to five hours.) Aim for night sleep to contain a stretch of solid sleep of six hours (around four months) and eight to ten hours (by the first birthday).

3. NOW, START TO ORGANIZE HER DAY

Some kids go from *overtired to totally wired* really fast. And once they cross the line, they get revved even more and struggle against sleep. So check your wake/sleep diary and try to put your infant down thirty minutes *before* you think the yawning will start.

Then, set up a great bedtime routine. And don't forget that an early bedtime will boost your baby's sleep.

Use rumbly white noise for all sleep. Consider starting the sound before the bedtime routine (to get her in the mood to sleep). You might even use white noise during meals, if your baby is so distracted that she just nibbles during the day and doesn't eat enough to keep her satisfied at night.

Finally, here's one more tip. If despite your best sleep schedule your little one continues to wake with hunger during the night, try boosting her daytime calories and adding a *dream feed* to prevent night waking before it happens. (I'll talk more about this in chapter 8.)

Keepin' It Real: Be Consistent (Most of the Time)

Experts love to warn new parents, "Be consistent!"

This is the kind of advice that can drive new moms and dads nuts . . . because it's impossible to be totally consistent in real life. Sometimes you get stuck shopping at naptime. Or you get so busy you need to delay a meal for an extra hour. Or another child in your house demands attention right when your little one's nap-time arrives.

And that's just on a normal day! You may also need to bend the rules if your baby is ill. And if company comes, all bets are off.

So don't feel like you need to run your schedule like a Marine drill sergeant. But if you and your baby's other caregivers can stick reasonably close to a flexible timetable and regular routines, you'll all sleep better.

This is especially true at night, because responding to crying one night and holding back the next will accidentally teach your munchkin to cry more. ("I'm confused. Sometimes she comes when I yelp. Hmm . . . let me try it louder and harder!")

So try to be consistent . . . and predictable. Use dim lights, warm milk, the 5 S's, storybooks, and loveys . . . along with a touch of lavender . . . every night, and offer a few cues at naptime as well. Within weeks, you'll establish a pattern of great sleep that will last for years to come.

Crib Notes:
Reviewing *The Happiest Baby* Way

- Surprisingly, the best time to start your bedtime routine is in the *morning*! Infants who get sunlight and walks outside during the day (and whose nursing moms avoid stimulants, like dark chocolate) sleep much better at night.

- Start giving you infant's brain some signals an hour before bedtime—dim lights, soft white noise, no roughhousing, no TV—that sleepy-time is coming.

- You can continue to use swaddling—even if your infant has begun rolling over—as long as you secure her in a *fully reclined* swing or a *fully reclined* infant seat.

- As the months pass, white noise becomes one of the most important sleep cues. It is key for helping your infant fall asleep after you wean the swaddling. And it will help her stay asleep despite outside noises and lights and discomforts like teething and tummy grumbling.

- Swinging—for naps and night sleep—continues to be a big help for the 5 to 15 percent of infants who are motion lovers.

- The *wake-and-sleep* technique is the key to building your infant's self-soothing skill and resisting the negative influence of the wrong sleep cues.

## CHAPTER EIGHT

Helping Your Infant Stay Asleep: Three to Twelve Months

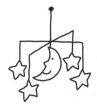

KEY POINTS:

★ Like struggles falling asleep, popping awake at night can happen when your little one is too revved up; something's disturbing her (teething, etc.); she's learned the wrong sleep cues; or she's going down too early (or too late).

★ You can gently reduce night feedings and boost sleep—even with bed-sharing babies—by increasing daytime calories (with *cluster feeds* and *dream feeds*) or using little techniques like the "Owie" trick.

★ New issues like teething and constipation can shatter your infant's sleep. But you can ease these pains—and many others—with some simple, natural, budget-friendly solutions.

★ For some kids, sleep training is a necessity. The *longer-and-longer* approach is a gentler alternative, or you can consider the *no-tears* method of *pick up/put down*!

If your baby is beautiful and perfect, never cries or fusses, sleeps on schedule and burps on demand, an angel all the time, you're the grandma.

—THERESA BLOOMINGDALE

Nighttime Cries—a Never-Ending Story?

Wahhhhh! Wahhhhh!

Night crying pulls on our heartstrings. And of course, we often jump right up because we don't want the entire household to wake (and we hope to lull our little one back to sleep before he fully wakes).

Night waking is *the* biggest sleep complaint of a baby's first year. About 25 percent of five-month-olds can't sleep six hours in a row. And frequent night wakers end up receiving one and a half hours less sleep overall!

New Zealand researcher Jacqueline Henderson and her colleagues had moms track their babies' sleep patterns. They found that:

■ **50 percent of three-month-olds slept five hours straight (not bad).**

■ **50 percent of five-month-olds slept eight hours, from 10 P.M. to 6 A.M. (jackpot!).**

■ **15 percent of infants couldn't even sleep five hours straight by their first birthday!**

So don't just wait for your five-month-old's sleep to fall into place on its own. A Canadian study found that a third of five-month-olds who woke at night still couldn't manage six hours of unbroken sleep at two and a half years of age!

Luckily, there are some very effective ways to stretch this time. First, follow the tips in the last chapter for establishing a calming bedtime (and prebedtime routine). Use a strong, rumbly white noise all night long, and help your sweetie learn to self-soothe by providing cues that don't involve your presence.

But the most important key to helping your infant sleep through the night is to know why she's waking.

Why Infants Wake at Night

If your infant is past five months and is still waking during the night (between midnight and 6 A.M.), you should consider whether she might be waking because of one of these four common problems:

- She's overexcited.

- Something's bugging her (including hunger).

- She's learned too many wrong habits and not enough good sleep cues.

- Your bedtime timing is off (it's too early, too late, or too irregular).

Does that list sound familiar? Not surprisingly, these are exactly the same reasons infants fight *falling* asleep.

Curb Her Enthusiasm for Bedtime Excitement

A baby who's bouncing off the walls at bedtime is more likely to wake you up at 2 A.M. as well. Luckily, this problem is pretty easy to resolve.

Spend the last hour before bedtime in quiet play, with the house lights dimmed, the TV and music off, and the white noise on. Also, avoid giving your infant any caffeine directly or through breast milk (see page 14). Of course, make sure you have a great sleep routine in place, too (see chapter 7).

Prevent and Soothe Disturbances

Jane says, "Zoe just turned five months old and has started waking at 2 A.M. again. She cries to eat, but then wants to play! We still swaddle her with one arm out and use ocean wave sounds, but now I also have to bounce her on her side for twenty to thirty minutes to get her back to sleep."

As I've mentioned earlier, your infant's sleep may be disrupted by *outside commotions* like bright lights or daddy's snoring—or by *inside discomforts* like teething, hunger, stuffy nose, and constipation.

And when she's roused, her discomfort or desires (like her love of social contact) may cause her to awaken completely and call for her favorite buddy and playmate . . . you!

Your best hope of masking these disturbances and guiding your groggy little sheep back to sleep is with *strong* white noise. Hissy fans and ocean waves may have worked during the first few months, but they often fail to soothe older infants with greater curiosity and bigger discomforts.

So make sure you use harsh, rumbling white noise, as loud as a shower, for all naps and nights. And if your infant is still waking, cover bright lights (put a towel over VCRs and clock radios, put dark shades on windows, and dim the hall light outside her door). Make sure the room isn't too hot or cold, and use a humidifier if the room is very dry or her nose is stuffy.

Of course, one of the biggest disturbances at this age is hunger. Your little one may be so distracted during the day that she forgets to eat and only realizes she's famished after the lights are out. Or she may eat all day and *still* be hungry at night because she's in the middle of a growth spurt.

Either way, there are a few ways to manage nighttime hunger so your little buddy is getting all the nourishment she needs . . . during the more agreeable daytime hours.

Feed Your Baby for Sleep Success

Heidi, mom of five-month-old Caden, said he suddenly went from perfect sleep to "A Nightmare on Elm Street"!

"Two weeks ago," she said, "we started rice cereal, then apples, bananas, and avocado. He eats two meals a day, midmorning and then around 7 P.M. Then he gets a bath, and he's down by 8 P.M. at the latest. But now, every two hours he cries until I come. The minute I pick him up he's totally happy, but he tears at my shirt and wants a big serving of his milkie. Then he's back asleep, but just for two hours!"

Heidi added, "I know he's exhausted because his naps went from one hour to two hours long, three times a day. And he's crankier, too."

Fortunately, it was pretty easy to get Caden back on track. I had Heidi totally stop the food during the day, offer the breast every two hours, and wake her little boy up at 11 P.M. for a dream feed. In two days, he was back to sleeping all night long.

As I've explained, sleeping and feeding just go together. We all get drowsy after a rich, warm meal. But most babies outgrow the *need* for middle-of-the-night meals by four to six months. So why do some, like Caden, suddenly start waking up again at 2 A.M. starving? Here are the top reasons.

They're eating diet food. Few things are as much fun as spooning pureed carrots into your baby's eager mouth. But the best source of nutrition for the first year isn't low-cal solid food like carrots or rice; it's high-cal milk. That's why Caden kept waking. He was filling up all day on salad bar cuisine: tasty and fun, but definitely diet food.

They're too nosy. Some infants are so distracted during the day that they just snack or skip some feedings altogether. Then, when they wake during the boring stillness of the night, they suddenly notice they're ravenously hungry.

It's a growth spurt. Remember that sudden surge in growth during your teens? Well, your infant will go through many growth spurts through the first year. He'll get so hungry that he'll pop awake during light sleep to chow down.

No matter what the cause, the best way to lessen hunger at night is . . . more milk during the day.

A Simple Solution: *Cluster* and *Dream Feeds*

If your baby wakes up hungry each night, besides boosting her daytime milk it makes sense to boost her evening calories. (Think of it like topping off the gas tank of your car by filling it to the brim.) Two classic ways to do this are *cluster feeds* and *dream feeds*.

Cluster feeds are a series of quick milky meals given every one to two hours from 4 P.M. to bedtime. They're meant to load your baby's system with calories to keep her *well stocked* with nutrition through the night.

Some doctors warn parents not to overfeed babies for fear that the milk might back up and cause colicky pain. But this is nonsense. The women in the !Kung tribe in Southern Africa feed their babies three or four times an hour, and their babies rarely—if ever—have colic.

So if your baby starts crying sixty minutes after a feeding, calm her with the *5 S*'s and then see how she acts. If she's opening her mouth and searching for a nipple, give a little more milk to make her tummy happy!

A *dream feed,* which I talked about earlier, is when you wake a *sleeping* baby to give her an extra feed. Research shows that sneaking in one more feed between 10 P.M. and midnight reduces night waking among three-month-olds . . . and it works great for older infants, too!

To do this, wake your wee one at around 11 P.M. and encourage her to nurse (five to ten minutes on one side, and the rest on the other side). Make sure when you put her down again, that you do the quick *wake-and-sleep* trick (see page 88).

If she has a hard time waking for the *dream feed*, change her diaper, tickle her toes, or cool her head with a wet washcloth to get her aroused enough to eat.

Dream feeds are great for your infant because:

- She'll get the extra calories she needs to sleep better.

- The meal's at a convenient time (so *you* sleep longer).

- The feeding is *not* in response to her crying (which would only *reward* the waking and end up encouraging more night feeding!).

- She'll eat less during the night and therefore be hungrier in the morning, which will boost her daytime eating.

If your baby continues to wake at 3:30 A.M. in spite of the *dream feed* and strong, rumbly white noise, consider setting your alarm to give one more *dream feed* at 3 A.M. The idea is to wake her *before* she wakes you so you're giving her the nourishment she needs, but not rewarding her for waking and crying.

If you have to do this early-morning *dream feed*, make sure you *give a little less milk*. If you're nursing, just feed on one side. If you're bottle-feeding, add double the amount of water the formula directions suggest (just for this one feeding) for a few days. Don't talk or cuddle too much. You want to be loving, but not to make her think it's time to play.

Every three days, reduce the 3 A.M. feed a little more by giving shorter feeds at the breast or putting more water in the formula. If you're breast-feeding, your breasts will quickly learn to make less milk at night and more during the day.

The goal: Give enough milk to get her back to sleep, but not so much that she eats less during the day.

Here are some extra tips:

- If your baby only eats one or two ounces at the 3 A.M. feed, try upping her calories a bit during the day and see if you can stop her middle-of-the-night munchies.

- If you're planning on giving a *dream feed* but your baby wakes up right before it was scheduled, it's okay to feed her and then move the feeding a little earlier the next night.

- If you're worried your baby's not getting enough milk, weigh her at your doctor's office to make sure she's growing normally.

Sleepytime Land Mines: Illness, Teething, and More

As you know, when your little robin is in the light part of her sleep cycle (right before taking another dive into deep slumber), an illness or physical discomfort can pop her back awake. Chances are high that sooner or later you'll have to deal with one of these sleep disruptors:

- Colds
- Snoring
- Teething
- Constipation

Earlier I gave you some advice on dealing with breathing problems and colds (see page 106). Those tips still work with older infants. (You can stop making visitors put on T-shirts over their clothes after three months, but it's still a good idea to have family members change their clothing after school or work—to stop germs from sneaking in—and they should all get their immunizations.)

And here's some additional (and important) advice about colds. When your cutie has the sniffles, don't give her:

- **Over-the-counter zinc nose drops or spray (it may damage the nerves and hurt your baby's ability to smell).**

- **Vicks VapoRub, if your infant is under two years of age (it can get into the eyes and be very irritating).**

- **Honey in any form before your child's first birthday (it can cause a potentially fatal illness called infant botulism).**

Also, make sure your infant is up to date with all *her* shots, including influenza. The flu is very common and easy for you to bring home. But it's *not* easy to fight off. In fact, it causes tens of thousands of hospitalizations and deaths among children under one year of age.

Now, let's look at the other sleep stealers that can arrive on the scene at this stage.

Snoring? Hmm . . . Not So Cute!

Does your infant sleep with his mouth open? Or snore? Or wake with an abrupt, loud snort? These behaviors may seem funny, but they could all be signs of sleep-disordered breathing, or SDB (also called obstructive sleep apnea)—a serious, but treatable, problem.

If your infant snores or chokes at night, try relieving his breathing with a cool mist humidifier and placing a folded towel *under* the mattress, to raise his head two to three inches. But if the noisy breathing continues, call your health-care provider for advice. (For more information on this problem, see pages 322–27.)

Head Banging: What's Up with That?

Little Quinn loved white noise and his nighttime bottle of milk. Initially, he settled down easily with the help of these sleep cues. But at nine months, he started to do something very bizarre: banging his head against the side of his crib!

Quinn would get up in the crawling position and go "bang—bang—bang" for ten minutes as he settled into sleep. This worried his parents, Kristin and Cory, because Quinn was developing a thick knot right above his left eye, where his forehead whacked the wooden bars.

Sound odd? Actually, head banging is pretty common from six months to three years—especially among boys. It often goes along with head rolling (from side to side) or humming. It never causes bleeding or any serious type of injury, but it can leave a bump that lasts for months (but goes away eventually). And it can be so strong that it actually makes the crib bang against the wall . . . or walk across the floor!

This form of rhythmic rocking is sort of a cousin of the 5 S's. It helps infants ignore things like outside noises or teething pain and may also help a child deal with worries or calm down from the day's exciting events . . . or relax him right before a big developmental leap (like walking).

There are several things you can do to try to end head banging:

- Replace exciting play and DVDs before bed with thirty minutes of calm, low-sensation play (dim lights, white noise, massage, rocking, singing, etc.).

- Lengthen your baby's bedtime routine by fifteen to thirty minutes.

Teething: It's Uncomfortable Growing Up

For centuries, grandmas and doctors have chalked up night
waking to teething pain. There's no question, teething can make
gums throb—and make your child want to bite on *everything* to
help push the tooth through the surface.

But is this really pain, or just discomfort? In truth, teething
happens—on and off—for many months. So the pain can't be so
bad, or all kids would be up every night for months. Besides, most
kids show no pain during the day.

In short, teething is usually just an annoyance: easy to ignore
during the day, but a bit more bothersome when lying flat in a
dark, quiet room.

The good news is that a little lovey and good, rumbly white
noise are usually all you need to distract your baby and help her
sleep right though crummy-feeling gums.

However, if you think discomfort is keeping your child awake,
ask your doctor about giving ibuprofen or acetaminophen thirty
minutes before bed (it takes a little time to work). And while
you're waiting for the medicine to work, let your munchkin chew
on a washcloth whose corner was dipped in apple juice and then
frozen.

The Poop Alarm Clock

Nighttime pooping can really disturb your infant's sleep, especially if he has to strain and struggle because of constipation.

Your baby's poops should never be hard little pellets or big pieces that strain or tear the anus. And while breast-fed babies may go days between *soft* poops during the first few months, all older infants should have soft poops at least once a day.

If you're concerned that hard, infrequent stools are making your guy grunt, wiggle, and wake at night, ask your doctor about changing his formula or softening the blockage with a suppository or an ounce of *organic* adult prune juice or fresh aloe vera juice mixed into two or three ounces of breast milk or formula every morning. (Give it a couple of days to work.)

Say "Good-Bye" to Old Habits and "Hello" to Great Sleep Cues

When eleven-month-old Gianni began waking two or three times a night, Gina felt a little guilty because the problem started right after she started back at work and enrolled him in day care. But two weeks later, she was exhausted. The only way she could get him back down was to nurse him and let him doze off on her chest, which was destroying her sleep.

Poor sleep habits are definitely the eight-hundred-pound *stuffed* gorilla in the bedroom of night-waking children.

Soothing babies—all night—with bed-sharing, rocking, and breast milk snacks seems totally reasonable. After all, parents have used them for thousands of years . . . and they definitely help babies fall asleep! No wonder so many parents do them, as you can see in the following table:

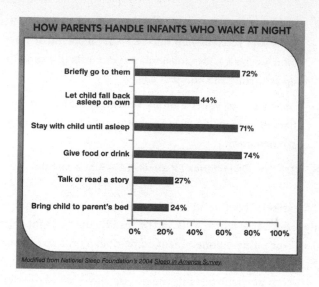

HOW PARENTS HANDLE INFANTS WHO WAKE AT NIGHT

Briefly go to them	72%
Let child fall back asleep on own	44%
Stay with child until asleep	71%
Give food or drink	74%
Talk or read a story	27%
Bring child to parent's bed	24%

0% 20% 40% 60% 80% 100%

Modified from National Sleep Foundation's 2004 Sleep in America Survey.

However, research shows that infants who are rocked, cuddled, and fed every time they wake may not learn how to fall back to sleep without help. So while all this coziness may speed your baby's return to slumber in the short term, it may also start an exhausting cycle: Waking ⇒ more bed-sharing ⇒ more waking ⇒ more bed-sharing.

The good news is that there's a way for you to enjoy this beautiful cuddling while simultaneously strengthening your baby's ability to self-soothe!

Love Nursing, but Ready to Sleep Longer?

After four months, you can start reducing nighttime nursing, yet continue daytime nursing. Here's how:

- Boost daytime calories by reducing mealtime distractions, using *dream feeds,* and trying the other steps I've just described.

- Use a strong, rumbly white noise for all naps and nights.

- Use the *wake-and-sleep* technique for all sleep times.

- Have your sweetie sleep next to his dad so he doesn't smell the sweet scent of your milk. Or wear a couple of T-shirts (and maybe a body stocking!) so your little guy can't just pull up your shirt and nurse at will.

- Shush or rock your infant back to sleep instead of nursing him. (But again, be sure to gently jostle him awake when you put him down.)

- Try the "Owie!" trick I'll describe in just a minute.

Of course, if your child is ill, stressed, or really hungry, it's fine to give him some warm milk in the middle of the night (just a few ounces—or nurse on one breast so he doesn't fill up so much that he has less appetite in the morning).

Weaning at night doesn't mean you have to wean during the day. The breasts have the *amazing* ability to turn off milk production at night and turn it back on in daytime. But when you start night weaning, always pump off one to two ounces—just enough to relieve pressure and prevent mastitis—at bedtime and again during the night, if you wake up with full breasts. If you pump more than that, your breasts will get confused and continue overproducing at night.

As with any plan, expect some backsliding during periods of stress (illness, travel, etc.) when your little one's need for soothing may increase for a few nights. If he has trouble giving up the nursing, just repeat the weaning process again.

Bed-Sharing? Yes! You Can Cuddle and Still Reduce Night Nursing

Melbourne's leading child sleep researcher, Dr. Harriet Hiscock, notes that parents who struggle with poor infant sleep usually bed-share and breast-feed. There's really no mystery to this; infants quickly learn that a few squawks gets them cozy sucking and a tummyful of milk. Like my friend Dana says, "If I had delicious cake in bed next to me, I'd wake and nibble all night, too."

Of course, setting limits when you're bed-sharing is tough because:

- You're tired.

- You want your baby to be happy and fall back asleep fast.

- It's your job and joy to feed your baby.

- You don't want to disturb your partner.

One way you can continue bed-sharing, yet still wean the night nursing, is with the "Owie!" trick.

The "Owie!" Trick

For months, Helena and Bill had loved snuggling with eleven-month-old Hanna all through the night. But while Bill could snore away the night, Helena was still waking every three hours to nurse. The divine Ms. Hanna wasn't superhungry; she just took a few gulps and drifted right back out. Helena, on the other hand, often needed twenty to thirty minutes to fall back asleep.

I suggested that Helena try a slightly sneaky approach:

1. Ramp up Hanna's calories during the day.

2. Teach her the meaning of "Owie!" by using it several times a day whenever she banged herself.

3. Teach her that Band-Aids go on owies and make them better. ("Yea! All better!")

4. At bedtime, put on the white noise, nurse, and then cover up with a couple of shirts and do the normal routine.

5. Once in bed, Helena should point to her breasts and whine to Hanna, "Owie! Owie! Owie!" and stick a Band-Aid on the T-shirt over each breast.

6. When Hanna wakes to nurse, Helena should point to the Band-Aid, saying, "Owie! Owie!," then give her to Bill to comfort for a few minutes.

Helena and Bill planned to give Hanna a bottle of pumped breast milk if she kept crying. But that first night, she woke twice and was comforted with just five minutes of cuddling. The second night was the same. And by the third night, she was sleeping all the way through!

Weaning the 5 S's

Up to now, the 5 S's have been your best friends at bedtime. But just as children outgrow their need for training wheels, kids outgrow the sleep cues that were so important to them as babies.

Since half of all four-month-olds sleep six to eight hours straight, that's a reasonable time to *begin* weaning your baby off a couple of her sleep cues. But this is not a race. It's a process that will take years. Sleep cues like blankies and teddys often go off to college with kids. (And as I mentioned earlier, we all use cues like darkness, quiet, or a favorite pillow to help our sleep.)

The first S parents phase out is all-night swinging. Most babies never need to sleep in the swing, but if you have a little motion lover who snoozed better when she was swinging all night, chances are she'll be ready to wean sometime between two and six months (although I did have one baby who needed the swing until nine months).

Once the swinging is over, the next S to go is swaddling. Since 80 percent of SIDS occurs before four months—and correct wrapping can prevent accidentally rolling to the risky stomach position—I recommend not weaning the swaddle until after four months. (Some infants need cozy wrapping for a few months longer.)

Most parents wean sucking on the pacifier at six to twelve months (it is fine to continue this longer—more about paci weaning on page 181). And finally, at twelve months or later, parents wean white noise (although many families continue to use white noise to promote sleep—through teething, vacations, new siblings, illnesses, and fears—for months or years to come).

Note: Side/stomach sleeping must be delayed until at least four months, but once started it never has to be weaned.

With those rough targets in mind, let's zoom in for a close look at the specifics for weaning these invaluable cues.

Weaning Swaddling

> *Ana and Jeff noted that their six-week-old son, Alex, slept eight to ten hours with white noise and snug swaddling. After his third month, they tried weaning him off the swaddling, but he started waking every two hours again. So Ana went back to the tight wrapping, and he slept through the night.*
>
> *By five months, Alex's personality blossomed. He loved the infant carrier but he insisted on facing out. Ana said, "He can't stand not seeing the action!" Jeff and Ana tried weaning the swaddling again, and this time it worked. After four days with one arm out, they stopped swaddling him altogether and Alex didn't even notice.*
>
> *Jeff said, "Now Alex can shoulder the responsibility of sleeping without being wrapped. After his 11 P.M. feeding, he's able to sleep eight hours straight, with just the help of his white noise."*

Swaddling is a great tool for the first few months. And some infants need it for six, eight, even ten months. These infants are just immature and jittery, and wrapping keeps them from accidentally startling themselves awake.

However, if your four-month-old is sleeping well, it's time to try weaning the swaddle. Here's how:

- **Wrap your baby with *one arm out*.**

- **If she continues to sleep well for a few nights, you can try stopping the swaddle completely (although I have cared for a few infants who still liked to be swaddled from the waist down).**

- **If she starts waking up and whacking herself in the face, restart swaddling and try the one-armed wrap again in a month, and every month thereafter until it works.**

Weaning swaddling is *much* harder if you're not using the right type of white noise all night. The new freedom from swaddling *plus* the stone silence of their room makes many infants wake up even more!

Weaning Sound

As you now are very well aware, rough white noise is key for improving your infant's naps and night sleep. (White noise that's too hissy or quiet may fail to work.) Use sound until *at least* your child's first birthday. Many parents continue it longer to help their toddlers or older kids sleep better . . . and even for themselves!

Don't worry that your child will become addicted. Sound is supereasy to wean. Just lower the volume little by little, over one to two weeks, and soon it will be history.

And if you ever want to restart the white noise on a trip or during an illness, you can just crank it back up, increasing the loudness over a few days.

Weaning Swinging

Mary Helen wrote me worried that she'd waited too long to wean her seven-and-a-half-month-old, Simon, out of the swing for his naps. I reassured her that even at that age the swing was fine, but I thought he might be able to be weaned if she used rough white noise.

I wrote, "After a week of letting him nap in the swing with the white noise, slow the swing down a step every three to four days until he'll nap in a nonmoving swing." Within two weeks, Simon was out of the swing.

Most infants sleep well enough with just swaddling and sound. But if your bouncy babe loves dancing and fast jiggling, sleeping in a swing may be absolutely indispensable.

If you use a swing for your infant's sleep, once she's sleeping well (usually by four to six months), simply reduce the swing's motion over a week or two—from fast to slow to off. Later on, you can try to wean the swaddling.

Weaning Sucking

The Academy of Pediatrics recommends a nighttime pacifier for the entire first year of life to protect against SIDS. But you may have to wean it sooner if:

- **Your infant has recurring ear infections. (Sucking hard on a pacifier may make these worse.)**
- **Your infant wakes each time the binky pops out.**

If you need to stop the paci early, be sure to use white noise all night. And after the six-month mark, consider swapping the pacifier for a cuddly lovey your sweetie can hold.

However, if your baby starts sucking his thumb, it's probably better to reintroduce the paci than allow your baby to get attached to his thumb. Thumb sucking pulls out the front teeth and pushes up the hard palate, causing much more extensive—and expensive—orthodontic problems than are seen with pacifiers.

Pick the Right Bedtime

If you've tried all these tricks and your drooly little friend is still waking at 3 A.M., consider the possibility that you have a bedtime scheduling problem. Three types of timing issues can lead to night waking:

- **Having a very irregular schedule**
- **Going to bed too early**
- **Going to bed too late**

The first point is pretty obvious. If you never know what time your boss will let you leave the office, it's really hard to plan dinner with your family. Similarly, if you keep changing the timing of her go-to-sleep routine, your baby never knows what to expect.

Early bedtimes can also cause problems. If your little bug falls asleep at 7 P.M., it's unlikely that she'll sleep all the way to 7 A.M. Instead, she'll probably wake for a couple of hours of play around 2 A.M.!

If you think bedtime may be too early:

- **Take a long walk in the bright sunlight every morning.**
- **Move the morning and noon feeds *later* by fifteen minutes (to nudge back the naps).**
- **Use rumbly white noise at all sleep periods.**
- **Keep your house lights bright until 7:30 P.M. (to delay melatonin release and sleepiness).**
- **Every three nights, move the start of your bedtime routine fifteen minutes *later*.**

If you're right and her bedtime was too early, you'll know soon. Within a week or two, her later bedtime routine should be faster and easier and she should have longer stretches of night sleep.

On the other hand, if the bedtime is too late, your infant will get so exhausted during the day that she falls asleep in the car while you're running errands with her. At bedtime she'll be cranky from overfatigue. And she'll have fitful sleep, whining and calling out every time her mind bobs into light sleep.

If you think bedtime may be too late:

- Take a long walk in the *bright sunlight* every morning.

- Move morning and noon feeds *earlier* by fifteen minutes (to slide forward the naps).

- An hour before bedtime, turn on rumbly white noise and dim your house lights (to enhance her melatonin release and sleepiness).

- Every three nights, move the start of your bedtime routine fifteen minutes *earlier* (*before* you see signs of fatigue).

Within a week or two, your sweet girl should act happier and sleep better . . . hopefully all through the night!

Early Birds: Little Ones Who Wake at the Crack of Dawn

Blake's early-morning wake-ups at eleven months of age were a mixed blessing for his dad. "It's great on weekdays," he told me. "Marnie gets to sleep in, and Blake and I have a quick stroll at dawn before I take off for work. But on the weekend? Hmmm, not so much. Couldn't the little guy at least sleep till seven on a Sunday?"

Most three- to twelve-month-olds wake around 7 A.M., but 10 percent pop up between 5 and 6 A.M. According to the Sleep in America poll, 21 percent of parents complain that their infants wake too early.

Early waking usually happens for one of four reasons. Your infant is:

- A little chickie who just likes to get up early.

- **Going to bed too early.**

- **Going to bed too late.**

- **Bothered by something.**

If your child is just an early bird who doesn't need much sleep, you better start going to bed earlier so you can adapt to her schedule!

However, if you think she may be waking early because her bedtime is too early or too late, follow the advice on pages 158–159 of this chapter for shifting an infant's bedtime.

If your child goes to bed at a normal time and you suspect she's waking due to morning disturbances (she's grouchy and overly tired during the day), try these tricks:

- **Darken the windows with heavy drapes if you think light is waking her.**

- **Use a strong white noise all night to mask distracting sounds.**

- **Boost her daytime calories and give a *dream feed* at midnight to reduce early-morning hunger.**

And of course, always check with her doctor if she seems to be awakened by breathing troubles (like snoring).

Sleep Training—the "Cry-It-Out" Controversy

Now, let's say that you've tried *every* trick in this chapter and the previous one, and nothing is working. It's rare, but it happens . . . and it's *not* because you're a bad parent! There are a handful of babies who are so spirited and strong-willed that they simply won't give in.

It's for this reason that most sleep experts recommend sleep training (which is really just a euphemism for letting your baby *cry herself to sleep*).

Now, I'll admit that *crying it out* can occasionally be needed—

but it shouldn't be your first approach. We can all get a door open by kicking it, but wouldn't you prefer just turning the knob?

So before you try sleep training, be sure you've followed *all* the steps outlined in the last two chapters for encouraging your infant to fall asleep and stay asleep. Also, make sure there are no new emotional traumas affecting her, such as new fears, big life changes (new school, house, or babysitter), seeing family fights, and so on.

When you've done all this, you can consider using sleep training . . . done correctly!

Three Methods of Infant Sleep Training

Over the past twenty years, experts have found three strategies to sleep train crying, resistant infants:

- **Cold turkey (also called *extinction*)**
- **Longer-and-longer (also called *graduated extinction*)**
- **Pick up / put down (also called *fading* or *camping out*)**

Here's a quick review, along with my recommendations on which method to choose.

Cold Turkey

In this method, you deposit your infant in bed, say "good night," and then leave, ignoring all cries until the morning.

The experts who promote this believe that babies must be allowed to cry to avoid spoiling. But there are many reasons why I would steer you away from this approach:

- **If your child vomits or accidentally injures herself, you'll have no idea till the morning.**
- **Your sudden absence may make her feel confused and abandoned.**
- **It may deeply upset a child with a sensitive or fearful**

- temperament, or one who's dealing with daytime stresses.

- ■ Some distraught, sensitive infants just can't calm without a bit of loving reassurance.

- ■ It's fundamentally disrespectful to ignore the cries of someone we love.

- ■ It makes parents feel terrible (anxious, guilty, frustrated, and incompetent).

Studies show that this approach *can* work, but it just seems wrong to spend all day building your tot's security by teaching that "Mommy and Daddy will help you" and then eroding that trust after the sun goes down.

Longer-and-Longer

Kyle was a rambunctious, persistent little guy. A real Mr. Personality! When he reached eight months, his parents, Neal and Laura, were exhausted and decided that it was finally time to sleep train him.

So Laura put him in bed awake and as long as his crying continued, she went in every fifteen minutes. She reassured him for thirty to sixty seconds at the crib side, but never picked him up.

"It was a miserable failure!" she recalled. "The first two nights, he cried for two hours!"

Then she changed her routine and began coming in more often (three, five, ten, and then every fifteen minutes) and only popping her head in for two seconds to say, "Sweet dreams, little man, I love you." And it worked: Kyle never cried longer than thirty minutes and was sleeping from 10 P.M. to 7 A.M. within three nights!

This is a kinder, gentler, more "graduated" (and more effective) version of *crying it out* popularized in the 1980s sleep classic, *Solve*

Your Child's Sleep Problems by Dr. Richard Ferber. (Some people still call this sleep training *Ferberizing*.)

If you're considering this route, first take a minute to think about your child's temperament.

Is she tenacious, stubborn, and spirited? If so, be prepared for her to push the limits harder and cry for an hour or more.

Is she shy, sensitive, and cautious? If so, she'll need more frequent visits (still brief) to reassure her that she isn't forgotten.

And if she's *very* sensitive or has experienced any recent traumas, fears, or major life changes, I strongly recommend skipping this approach and moving on to the next one (*pick up/put down*).

If you do choose this approach, here's how to do it. After your full bedtime routine:

- **Put your baby in bed, turn on the white noise, say "Night-night" and leave the room.**

- **Open the door again after three minutes of crying. (Keep the bright hall light off and just have a night-light in the room.)**

- **Pop your head in the room for a few seconds (long enough to see if she's hurt or vomited). Say something sweet and loving, like "Night-night, night-night. I'll kiss you in the morning light," then leave.**

- **If her crying continues, return in five minutes and repeat the same quick check and leave. If it still persists, return in ten minutes, and then every fifteen minutes, to repeat the exact same message. (That's why this approach is called *longer-and-longer*.)**

You might worry that showing your face will only make your infant cry more. But the goal is to teach her that you love her and care about her feelings, *but* that you've made a clear decision not to come in and relent to her unreasonable demand.

Resist the temptation to stay too long. For most (although not all) babies, talking more and coming closer to the crib only causes *more* crying. That's because (1) it's frustrating (like holding a bag of potato chips in front of a hungry child and giving her only one) and (2) it's a tease (it raises her hopes that the crying is working, only to dash them when you walk out of the room).

Expect the first night to be rough. You'll have to toughen your heart a little. And during any middle-of-the-night waking, you'll need to repeat this whole process.

Usually the second night is the same or a little worse, but the third night is much better. And by the fourth night, most infants fall asleep quickly and sleep until morning.

(Note: Your infant may throw you a curveball and go back to crying for an hour on the third or fourth night. This may happen if she's ill or supertenacious or if you are inconsistent with your responses—talking too much, coming too close, or staying too long. If you find yourself in this situation, don't lose faith. Just quickly check to make sure your baby is okay and stick to the routine.)

Don't use *longer-and-longer* for naps. Naps are so short that irritated infants sometimes cry the whole time and end up miserable for the rest of the day. Fortunately, once night sleep is well established, naps automatically get better. So just continue your flexible nap schedule and use the lovey and strong white noise.

Here are some extra hints for success:

- **Make sure you and your partner fully agree on the plan.**

- **Throw away the idea that letting your baby cry makes you a bad parent (that's totally false). If you've created a stellar bedtime routine and you've offered all the right cues, and you're *still* not getting any sleep, gentle sleep training can make everyone happier.**

- **Start your sleep training on a weekend or a day off so you can rest up the next day.**

- **If your tot is persistent, defiant, independent, and strong-**

willed, don't be surprised if the first night's crying goes on for thirty to sixty minutes . . . or more!

- If your child shares a bedroom with a sibling, let your older child sleep in your room or the living room until the training is over. And use white noise with your older child so he can't hear the crying.

- If you're in a one-bedroom apartment, keep your baby in the bedroom—but *you* should sleep in the living room until the training is completed.

- Warn your neighbors about your plans, so they don't get worried and call the police! (Offer to loan your neighbors a white noise CD to help them sleep through the crying.)

- Since you won't be going to see your baby as often to change her, make sure she has a good thick layer of cream on her bottom to protect her skin.

- Some pains do throb more when we lie down. So if you think your little one might have teething pain, ask your doctor if it's okay to give a little medicine thirty minutes before bedtime.

Note: If you feel like you're crumbling after thirty minutes of crying and you need to go and rescue your angel, *you can.* You should always follow your instincts. But remember, the more inconsistent you are, the more you'll accidentally teach her that screaming will get her the things she wants.

Extinction Bursts—*Crying It Out* Often Gets Worse Before It Gets Better!

Your rapid responses over the first three to six months actually teach your child exactly how hard to cry to get you into the room fast. That's good, because you want your infant to know how to get you when he really, really needs you.

Unfortunately, like the boy who cried wolf, some older infants abuse their smoke-alarm-like scream power to summon their parents even when it's not an urgent matter. And what's worse, they may get locked into their screaming if their parents don't come fast. (This is especially likely to happen when they're overtired and cranky.)

So if you decide to do the *longer-and-longer* sleep training, don't be shocked if on the first night, your little lovebug screams louder and harder than he's ever screamed before. In fact, this escalation is totally normal for one to two nights.

Psychologists call this an *extinction burst*—a burst of crying that occurs before the behavior ends (or as they say in psych lingo, *is made extinct*).

It will probably take two to four days for your little snookie to learn that there's now an exception to the "you cry—I'll come" rule you've spent the past four months teaching him. So brace yourself for a wild ride, but remember that it won't last long.

Pick Up/Put Down—the No-Tears Solution

Mona, the mom of ten-month-old Lulu, was advised to place her infant awake into the crib and to sit in the room in a chair away from the crib but where Lulu could see her. She also was told to just keep saying reassuring words until Lulu fell asleep.

Lulu shrieked and wailed pitifully, stretching her arms out between the bars. She kept falling into the bars and crying even more. Mona felt just terrible. After forty-five minutes, she gave up and gathered her sobbing little princess into her arms to rock her to sleep.

Unfortunately, Mona got inaccurate advice about the method called *pick up/put down*. The *correct* way to use this gentle approach is to respond to any fussing, even taking your infant from bed if needed. Over several nights, you gradually respond less and less until you're just sitting quietly a little distance away as she settles into sleep.

Pick up/put down (also called *fading*) is what I recommend to parents who want to avoid any bedtime crying. It takes longer (thirty to ninety minutes per night) and more days (four to fourteen), but it can be very effective and less traumatic. It's especially helpful for infants who are going through lots of changes in their lives or who tend to be anxious or fearful.

Here's the drill:

- Place your little one in the crib (waking her if she's already asleep).

- If she cries, pick her up and comfort her. Acknowledge her feelings in quiet tones: "I know, I know, honey. You say, 'Mommy, pick me up now!' It's hard falling asleep, huh, sweet pea?"

- Once she calms, put her down again.

- If she cries, pick her up . . . and repeat this cycle *over and over*.

- Do as little rocking, patting, talking, or feeding as you can, to reduce her dependence on these more demanding cues.

This approach takes a lot of patience. The first few nights, you may have to pick her up and put her down fifty times!

As always, use a rough white noise for all naps and nighttime sleeping and encourage the use of a lovey. And plan this training when you're off the next day, so you can sleep late or nap.

Also, be aware that *pick up/put down* doesn't work well if:

- **You offer too big a reward (talking, playing, nursing) every time you pick her up.**

- **Your infant has a tenacious, determined temperament and just won't give up. (That's when you might have to go back to the *longer-and-longer* technique.)**

With the *cold turkey* and *longer-and-longer* approaches, *you* set the bedtime you want. But with *pick up/put down*, you start your routine at your child's natural sleep-time and then move it earlier by fifteen minutes every other night until you have it where you want it.

What If Your Infant Vomits During Sleep Training?

A mom from a small island in South Korea wrote, "Our daughter, Na-young, is now eight months old. For about one month she has been waking up every hour, and she cries until she is held. If I sleep with her in my arms, she'll go at least two hours, but then I don't get any sleep. I tried to let her just cry, but every time I do that she gags terribly and vomits."

Some babies cry so hard that their abdominal muscles tighten and accidentally expel the entire contents of the stomach.

Naturally, when that happens, it's easy to feel terribly guilty. And we want to immediately clean and comfort our babies before laying them down again.

But this is a little tricky, because giving too much cuddly

attention after your baby vomits may inadvertently teach him that vomiting is a quick way to get the attention he wants.

So what should you do if your baby vomits during the first night of sleep training?

Quickly clean him off, with as little cuddling and soothing talk as possible. Check to make sure he's not sick, change his crib sheet and PJs, and then place him back down. Then say "night-night" and start the routine over again from the beginning. If you do any more than that, there's a risk that you'll accidentally encourage the vomiting to become a habit.

Sleep Training If You and Your Tyke Share the Same Bedroom

It's possible to sleep train an infant who's sleeping in the same room as you, but it's definitely tough.

When your infant can see you, she'll naturally keep trying and trying to get you to pick her up. That's why—if at all possible—I recommend that you and your partner sleep in the living room and keep your infant in the bedroom while you're doing the training. Or consider using the *pick up/put down* method instead of *longer-and-longer*.

But if you have no other choice, here are a few tips to help you manage the training with your baby in your room:

- Put a screen or sheet across the room so she can't see you.
- Work extrahard beforehand to get her interested in a lovey.
- Use strong white noise so she doesn't hear you breathing, talking, or snoring (and so her cries will be less upsetting to you).
- Consider beginning her sleep training *during naps.* This may help her respond faster when you introduce the new system at night.

Retraining: Helping Infants After They Backslide

Don't be shocked if you have to sleep train your infant again two months after you did it the first time. Infants can slide back into their old waking pattern for many different reasons, including illness, travel (and time zone changes), scary experiences, or major life changes.

Fortunately, this type of backsliding may correct itself in a few days. However, if the problem doesn't get better fast, just go back to your step-by-step sleep-training routine. It's usually faster and easier each time you do it.

Be Aware—Depression Still Can Lurk

I hope you haven't had to endure the flood of anxious worries and feelings of isolation that typify postpartum depression (PPD). However, it's important to be aware that although PPD usually occurs shortly after birth, it can creep up like a shadow many months later and last for months or even years. So if you're feeling sad, anxious, or isolated, don't hesitate to ask for help.

And remember that getting your infant's sleep under control can be hugely effective in reducing your depression. One group of researchers reported a 45 percent drop in depression scores after mothers learned how to boost their babies' sleep.

Getting There . . . by Different Roads

If there's anything I know after decades of baby watching, it's that no two infants are alike. That's why I've offered a variety of different approaches you can use to help your little one sleep longer and better.

In most cases, a great sleep routine and powerful cues like loveys and white noise do the trick. But don't feel guilty if they don't! Your spirited or sensitive child may push the envelope for years to come, and you'll often need to take extra steps to keep her on track. In this case, that might mean *pick up/put down* or *longer-and-longer*.

So just keep at it, and sooner or later you'll hit the jackpot. In my experience, perseverance pays off . . . and eventually, you'll get the good night's sleep you deserve!

Crib Notes: Reviewing *The Happiest Baby* Way

- White noise—*rough, rumbly,* and as loud as a shower—masks the minor disturbances that commonly wake infants (like passing trucks, throbbing gums, mild hunger, and tummy rumbles) and quickly guide them back to sleep.

- Hissy fans and ocean waves often fail to boost sleep because they aren't rough and rumbly enough.

- Use the *wake-and-sleep* technique to wean your infant from unwanted sleep cues (like nighttime feeds and needing to be rocked to sleep).

- The "Owie!" trick is a slightly sneaky way to wean nighttime nursing. It's based on Band-Aids . . . and your infant's growing sense of empathy.

- The *5 S*'s are great bedtime friends, but between three and twelve months you will slowly phase them out, except for white noise.

- The order of weaning the *5 S*'s is usually swinging first, then swaddling, sucking, and finally whooshy sound.

- White noise also makes sleep training easier and more successful.

## CHAPTER NINE

Q&A: Common Questions About Infants' Sleep: Three to Twelve Months

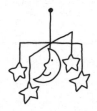

1. Our five-month-old has bowel movements in her sleep. Should I wake her to change the diaper even though it might wake her up again?

Babies frequently pee and even poop during the night. And usually you won't hear when it occurs, so it is hard to know exactly when a diaper needs to be changed.

So before you tuck her in, always put a nice layer of protection on her bottom (cocoa butter or zinc oxide is nice; avoid creams with artificial ingredients like fragrance, parabens, and petrochemicals).

But if you hear a BM—which often happens during or shortly

after eating—of course you should change her diaper right away to prevent a rash.

And don't worry about getting her back to sleep. Your little bunny still has a full tummy of your warm milk and she's mildly "drunk" from that sweet meal. So just swaddle her back up, keep the white noise on, and rock her a little bit. She should fall back asleep in just a minute or two. That's the beauty of the S's: they let you place your infant back in bed awake, yet still help her glide back to sleep on her own.

2. Why is my ten-month-old so fussy when I take him to my mother-in-law's home?

After the six-month mark, infants become increasingly aware of the world around them and recognize what (and who) is familiar or foreign.

The changes between your home and your mother-in-law's that seem minor to you—like the different cribs, room lights, sheet textures, and even the strong odor of a perfumed fabric softener—may be *huge* to your baby. He'll probably spot *every* clue that he's no longer in his favorite place.

This is especially the case if your little guy is sensitive to other things in his life, like the lumpiness of his food or the scratchiness of his clothes.

So try to create as many similarities as possible between the two locations. Use the same loveys, decorations, night-lights, sheets, scents (a drop of lavender oil on the mattress can be useful), and—most important—the same rough white noise as you use at home.

3. Our doctor told us to stop night feeds, since our seven-month-old has hit twenty pounds. But he's still so hungry at night—what should we do?

Trust your instincts on this one! There are very few parenting laws that work for every child.

Twenty pounds is not a magic number. Some tots are tall, so they're still skinny at twenty pounds. Some kids go through growth spurts every few months, so even pudgy babies can be very hungry. And even eighteen-pound seven-month-olds can usually sleep through the night with just one *dream feed*.

If your little bruiser only snacks at night, he's probably just into the habit of night waking. Follow the advice in chapter 8 to help your infant sleep through the night.

However, if he eats all day and is *still* really hungry at night, he's probably having a real growth spurt. In that case, you might help him sleep better at night by:

- **Making sure he eats well during the day (lots of milk, not filling up on low-cal solids, and not distractedly snacking because of too much commotion around him).**
- **Doing *cluster feeds* in the evening and a *dream feed* at 11 P.M.**
- **Making sure you're putting him to bed at the right time; avoiding caffeine-like stimulants; protecting him from disturbances.**

4. When is it okay for my infant to sleep in the room alone with my toddler?

Toddlers can be very sweet with babies, but they just can't be expected to be cautious and protective. They have no idea about the fragility of infants.

I've had plenty of toddlers in my practice lovingly—but dangerously—offer their baby brothers and sisters crackers, metal trucks, pointy pens, and cuddly pillows.

So don't let your defenseless baby sleep in the same room as your marauding little tyke. Wait until your younger one can really protect herself, probably around her second birthday.

5. My child keeps losing the paci at night. Should I pin one to her shirt or leave a few in her crib?

It's fine to leave binkies in each corner of the bed. Point them out to your baby during the day (*"Oh! Look! Here's another paci over here!"*) to help her get used to finding them at night.

If that doesn't work or you want to make it even easier, you can get a paci with a little clamp that clips onto the PJs. That will keep it close by whenever she wants it. But never pin it on or use a ribbon to fasten it around her neck (this is a choking hazard).

And don't forget to use white noise and offer a silky blanket or cuddly teddy bear to encourage her to adopt a binky alternative that will be easier to manage and wean in the future.

6. I love nursing my eight-month-old, but when should I wean the nighttime feeds?

Many moms say that breast-feeding is one of the most wonderful experiences of parenting. And it's superhealthy for both your baby and you. So, as long as you and your husband are happy with the night nursing, there's no rush to wean.

However, if you need more sleep, your little friend is certainly old enough to go from 10 P.M. to 6 A.M. without a nursing. Just follow the weaning steps listed on page 175 . . . and don't forget to pump a little milk at night if you're feeling overly full.

7. My ten-month-old daughter stands in the crib but can't sit back down. (It's not so cute at 3 A.M.!) Any suggestions?

Your little girl is sending such a powerful message to her legs to straighten and stand that she's having a hard time reversing this message to tell her legs to relax, flex, and sit back down.

Fortunately, most babies learn leg bending pretty fast with a little practice. During the day, try these exercises:

- **Let her pull up on your fingers and then guide her back down by lowering your fingers.**

- Put your hands under her armpits and guide her up and down. Bring her to 90 percent standing, but then help her back down before her legs lock.

- In the crib, get her standing and then show her how to slide her hands down a little to make it easier to lower herself.

PART III

Sleep Solutions in the Toddler and Preschool Years: One to Five Years

Chapter 10 updates you on the big changes in your tot's verbal and mental abilities and teaches some special *Happiest Toddler* tips for building patience and cooperation that will help you create a wonderful bedtime (like the *Fast-Food Rule, Toddler-ese,* and *patience-stretching*). In addition, you'll learn why having a TV in your child's room increases sleep struggles and obesity, and how to move your tot from the crib to a bed.

Chapter 11 shows why the best bedtime routine actually starts . . . right after *breakfast*! You'll also learn new *toddler-perfect* sleep routines (like a *Beddy-Bye* book and *bedtime sweet talk*) and find out how to persuade your stubborn tyke to "get with the program" through family meetings, incentives, and simple, *no-cry* ways of sleep training like the *twinkle interruptus* trick and putting your toddler *on hold.*

Chapter 12 talks about common sleep disruptions as well as new ones—pinworms and growing pains—that can pop up at this age. I'll discuss how to wean nighttime nursing and bed-sharing and how to quell sleep-shattering fears. In addition, you'll get the lowdown on sleepwalking, night terrors, and nightmares.

Chapter 13 answers some of the most common sleep questions voiced by parents of toddlers and preschoolers.

## CHAPTER TEN

"Ready, Set . . . Go!" Welcome to the Hectic Life of Little Kids: One to Five Years

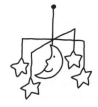

KEY POINTS:

- ★ Your toddler's brain is developing fast, but it's still immature and can make her act uncivilized—like a little *cave-girl*—when she gets upset.

- ★ Toddlers *love* running, dancing, and exploring— and they can be pretty rigid in their reactions to your requests—all of which can add up to rebellion at naps and bedtime!

- ★ Six fun *Happiest Toddler* techniques quickly boost your child's patience and cooperation in the daytime—leading to an easier time at tuck-in: the

Fast-Food Rule; Toddler-ese; patience-stretching; magic breathing; gossiping; and *playing the boob.*

★ **Toddlers sleep twelve to fourteen hours a day, but without a good sleep plan, half of them still wake up during the night and call for assistance.**

★ **Moving your toddler from crib to bed is easy with a little planning.**

★ **Poor sleep can have serious impacts on a young child's health.**

Can there be a creature on earth as adorable—and as trying—as a toddler?

—ANNE CASSIDY

Kid Stuff: What's Going On in Your Tot's Mind?

Toddlers never slow down . . . and neither do the changes going on inside them.

There's a *huge* increase in brain activity during these early years. Two-year-olds have twice as many busy, buzzing brain connections (synapses) as we do. No wonder they prance instead of walk and joyously squeal when they're happy. Three- and four-year-olds' energetic minds constantly compare and analyze things ("Your boobies are made out of pillows," or "Lie on my pillow, Mom; we'll look at my dreams together").

This enormous burst of brain maturation enables your little explorer to master skills that took our ancestors hundreds of thousands of years to develop—from walking and running to speaking, reading, joking, and even taking turns and using manners.

However, anyone who's hung out with young kids knows they're sweet and silly, but sometimes they also act totally *uncivilized!*

I don't mean to be disrespectful when I say this, but you have to admit they can be primitive. They bite, scratch, spit, and hit when upset. They're impatient and impulsive . . . and they pee anywhere they want! In fact, a huge part of your job during these early years is to teach your little *cave-kid* patience and manners.

Knowing a bit about the developmental leaps young kids make will help you understand why your tot struggles against sleep . . . and how to get him to love it. We'll take a closer look at these advances shortly—but first, let's see how tots of different temperaments handle the world.

Toddler Temperament: Little Kids with Big Personalities

Patient? Cautious? Moody? Supersensitive? Hyperactive? Like a flower opening in the spring, your tyke's temperament is revealing more of itself with each passing month.

Easy Kids

Easy kids bop through life on an even keel. Bumps and falls don't faze them much, and they take frustrations in stride. Many of them eat, sleep, and even poop at more or less the same time each day.

That's not to say easy kids never have meltdowns or act defiantly. But when things go wrong, easygoing children tend to shake it off and move on. ,

Cautious Kids

Eighteen-month-old Jesse was a very shy guy. His mom, Jody, said, "He only speaks four words, but he's a thinker. He practices things in his mind before he does them. At the park, Jesse spent weeks carefully watching kids crawl through a little tunnel. Then one day he tried it himself. After he did it once, he was so giddy that he did it twenty times in a row."

An easy child's first word is often a cheery "Hi!," but a cautious child's is often a worried "Bye!" He may timidly reserve his waves of farewell—until after your guests are out of the house and halfway to the street.

These tykes tend to trail their moms from room to room. One

of my eighteen-month-old patients was so clingy that her mom nicknamed her "Velcro."

Cautious kids are often overly sensitive to any little disturbance—teething, noises, hunger, strong odors, a stuffy nose, scratchy PJs, and so on. They frequently have trouble transitioning from the quiet of their parent's car into the buzz and bustle of the day-care center.

> *"Every morning at nursery school, Derek clings to me like plastic wrap for the first ten minutes," Tim said. He admitted, "I want to yell at him, 'Snap out of it!'"*

It's easy to run out of patience with an overly worried kid. But impatience *always* makes these toddlers more reluctant.

Cautious kids like Derek can be terrified if they feel pushed. Pressure these toddlers too much and their fears take twice as long to fade. But with months and months of gentle encouragement you'll definitely see your cautious child get increasingly confident—even brave.

And the bonus for parents of cautious kids is that when they grow up, their hesitant nature makes them less likely to race motorcycles, experiment with drugs, or gamble away their savings!

Spirited Kids

> *Elise said her fearless two-year-old was "100 percent ability and 0 percent judgment.*
>
> *"Spencer would go straight up to an axe murderer and say, 'Nice axe you got there!' He was in motion every waking second. His sister, Rosy, would just sit and study a toy for hours, but Spencer bounced like a Super Ball. That's why I would jump every time I heard the loudspeaker at Walmart announce, 'Hi, shoppers, we have a little boy . . .'"*

Spirited toddlers are wilder, nosier, and more rigid, active, defiant, impatient, stubborn, and impulsive than other kids. For them the "terrible twos" often start at fifteen months! Be prepared for tantrums . . . and don't be surprised if your headstrong child issues a defiant "No!" and crumples into tantrums and tirades when it's time for naps or bedtime (especially if he's overtired).

What's New in the Toddler Years? A Lot!

Whatever your tyke's temperament—easy, cautious, or spirited—she'll be undergoing big changes as she leaves babyhood behind. Here's a look at what kids this age are like.

Their Ability to Talk and Listen Skyrockets

Infants tell us what they want through smiles, cries, and grunts. But during the toddler years, your child's ability to communicate takes two huge steps forward, thanks to changes in both the right and left halves of his brain.

First, there's a surge of development in the right half—the part that controls gestures we make with our hands and face and that perfectly matches your little bub's tone of voice to his quickly shifting emotions.

You may have already noticed signs of this development, as he:

- **Points to things**
- **Uses sign language**
- **Gets more dramatic (using grins, frowns, hand flourishes, and changes of voice to show if he's happy, sad, frightened, frustrated, etc.)**

Second, as your child zips past his second and third birthdays, the left brain—the part that controls words, reasoning, patience, and self-control—gets a gush of growth boosting his ability to speak in words and sentences. (It's amazing how quickly kids go from barely babbling to being as tenacious as little courtroom lawyers . . . arguing why it's not fair to have to go to bed so early.)

They Love Activity!

Eighteen-month-old Trevor popped up like a jack-in-the-box every time he was put down for a nap. His mom said, "It's like telling Christopher Columbus to come in and take a nap. And, he's like, 'No way! I'm discovering America!' "

Once kids start walking, running, and climbing—look out! They get so jazzed by moving and exploring they forget their hunger, pee in their pants, and struggle like punch-drunk fighters against sleep.

Your young child is a little explorer who's interested in everything. When she hears conversation in another room, Ms. Nosy wants to investigate, so she doesn't miss a thing! (No wonder Curious George is such a toddler favorite.)

They Turn Into Little "Dr. No's"

Your toddler may often get quite rigid. We, too, can be pretty picky about wanting *our* pillow and *our* bed. But your toddler will sometimes be absolutely inflexible and insistent on doing things "just so"!

She may refuse to eat a cracker if it has a broken corner. Or make you read the same books every single night.

And this obsessive attitude usually gets even worse when your tyke is tired. You may have to kiss all the stuffed animals good night in exactly the right order . . . and start reading the book *all over again* if you accidentally skip a page.

Luckily, by three or four, your child will become more flexible (although she may still insist on wearing her favorite PJs to bed . . . every night!). By then, she will think you're funny if you make a "mistake," like singing "rock a bye baby" but inserting the word *birdie* for *baby*, or if you start reading a book on the last page.

They Love Routines!

Related to your little one's penchant for rigidity is her love of routines.

Doing the same routine every day may be boring to us, but for your toddler, routines are like safe little islands of predictability amid the chaos of the day. They are respite from the hard work tots do all day trying to understand all the new things that confront them. (Think of it like taking a tough test and suddenly coming upon a section of supereasy questions.)

Sometime before eighteen months, you'll notice that your tot is starting to show an interest in order. For example, she may like putting all the dinosaurs in one pile and the dolls in another.

And over the ensuing months, she'll start loving snack time, sharing circle at preschool, and singing silly songs. These all give structure to your tot's day and help her feel smart because she knows exactly what's about to happen.

Special Time: A Fab Routine That's Fast and Fun

You give your toddler *hours and hours* of playtime. So why does she get so demanding the minute you start cooking dinner?

Simple: *She's bored!* In past centuries, children's lives were a lot more interesting. They had tons of time outside playing with a fascinating mix of rocks, puddles, chickens, and kids.

But here's a fun little routine that will help make up for all that missing play: *special time*.

Once or twice a day, set aside five minutes to do anything your little buddy wants. You can even announce it with a peppy little song:

"It's Wendy's *special time*. Special, special, special . . . SPECIAL time!" Then set the timer and give her your undivided attention (no phones allowed!).

When the timer rings, say, "Aww . . . I'm so sorry, honey, special time is over . . . it was really fun . . . we'll have another special time a little later (or tomorrow)."

This time together wonderfully nourishes your toddler's self-confidence. ("If the beautiful queen of my house spends time *with just me* . . . I must really be special.")

Now, I know you're already spending tons of time playing with your child. But *special time* is different. This is a gift, a bite-sized bonus that's made extrayummy by the way you promote and announce it and by the undivided attention you give. (There are more tips on *special time* in the book *The Happiest Toddler on the Block*.)

Now that you know what's going on inside your young child's cute little head, here's a brief review of some surprisingly effective *The Happiest Toddler* techniques for having an easy toddler . . . even at bedtime.

Six Fun Steps to Boost Patience and Cooperation

As I noted earlier, your toddler's brain is zooming along, maturing more and more every week, but there will be times when emotional eruptions knock her back a million years into *cave-girl* mode. At those times, logic and reason may be a total flop, but a few other simple steps will make you much more successful.

When you combine win-win solutions with all of your bedtime sleep cues, you'll solve many sleep problems quickly. Here is a quick review of all the tricks you can use at this stage to get your little cub tucked in happily:

Build confidence during the day with *Toddler-ese, patience-stretching, magic breathing, gossiping, playing the boob,* sticker charts, role-playing, fairy tales, and a *Beddy-Bye* book.

Have thirty to sixty minutes of quiet time with the lights dimmed and the TV off before you start your routine. A warm bath and a massage can also relax your child.

Let your sweetie say good night to all the toys!

Use white noise, loveys, storybooks, lullabies, lavender, and *bedtime sweet talk* to help your child drift off. A pacifier is fine at this stage, too.

Offer compromises . . . both during the day and at night . . . so everyone can win.

Step 1: The "Fast-Food" Rule (FFR)—How to Connect With Your Upset Child

The rule for talking with people (tots included) is: *Whoever is feeling the most emotion (happiest, saddest, etc.) gets to speak first* (and gets an extralong turn). The other person listens and acknowledges the first person's feelings—just the way an employee at a fast-food restaurant repeats an order back to a customer before she gets to *her* agenda . . . asking for payment.

Note that to show your friend you *sincerely* care, it's *very* important for you to reflect a bit of her level of emotion in your tone of voice and gestures as you acknowledge her feelings. Reflect too little and you'll sound cold and removed; use too much and you sound over the top and hysterical.

As your friend starts to calm, *then* it becomes your turn to reassure, explain, give your reasons, offer a hug, find a compromise . . . or just sit together quietly.

You'll have a much easier time getting her to see *your* side if you first let her know that you see things from *her* side (even if you don't agree with her).

Step 2: "Toddler-ese"—Speaking Your Tot's Primitive Language

When adults get upset, we dial down the calm, logical left half of our brain and dial up the emotional right half. That's why frustration, fear, grief, and anger all make us less eloquent, less patient, less reasonable—in a word, more *primitive*. No wonder the name we give this brain drain is "going ape!"

But the brain's imbalance is even more exaggerated with toddlers.

Even on a good day, your toddler's left brain doesn't work that great. So when she gets upset, it dials almost completely off. That's why our little cave-kids don't just go ape . . . they go *Jurassic* on us—spitting, scratching, and throwing things at our heads!

So, when you are using the FFR, the more upset your child gets, the more basic—primitive—your phrases need to become. Fortunately, there's a way to communicate that will help you quickly connect with your little Neanderthal (and stop more than 50 percent of her tantrums in seconds): *Toddler-ese*.

Upset toddlers totally understand our caring messages when we stop our adult *left-brain* language (calm, wordy, long sentences) and translate it to a more *right-brain* language (remember that side of the brain is working fine). To do this, just convert what you want to say with these three steps:

- **Break it down into short phrases (one to four words).**
- **Repeat the phrases over and over (four to eight times).**
- **Use your gestures and tone of voice to mirror *a bit* (just one-third) of your child's upset.**

For example, when your little girl is upset, use this primal language to describe exactly what you see ("You're sad, sad, *sad!* Your ice cream fell! You are so, so sad!"). She may not understand all your words, but she can perfectly read your voice, face, and hand gestures.

Now, you may think this all sounds silly or like baby talk or that it sounds a bit unnatural. But I bet you're already using *Toddler-ese* . . . every single day!

Think about it. When your tyke proudly beams back at you after she struggles to the top of a little hill, would it feel more normal to calmly state, "Very good, sweetheart, Mother is proud," or to reflect her enthusiasm and applaud and chirp, "Yea! Yea! You did it! You did it! Wow! You did it all by yourself! Good job!"? Hey . . . that's *Toddler-ese*: short phrases, repetition, a bit of emotion.

Yet we often abandon *Toddler-ese* the minute our kid gets scared, mad, or sad. Suddenly, we either yell or try to calm her by acting overly calm ourselves. But that can make your toddler feel alone, like you don't understand or care about her upset . . . just when she needs a friend. (Sort of the way *you* might feel if your friend responded to your upset by immediately trying to *paper over* it by saying, "It's okay . . . It's okay . . . It's okay . . . It's okay," or flatly parroted your words—like some pseudopsychiatrist—"I can hear that was very frustrating for you.")

You'll need to practice *Toddler-ese* to get the hang of it. It can feel a little odd at first—but remember, you're already using it when your child is really happy. Many parents say the easiest way to learn this is to first use it when responding to *little* ups and downs. Then, gradually you can start using it for bigger upsets.

Toddler-ese isn't magic, and some upset kids will continue their outburst no matter what you say. But when done correctly, thirty seconds of *Toddler-ese* can calm over 50 percent of your cave-kid's meltdowns in seconds—even when she's overtired and fighting bedtime.

Step 3: "Patience-Stretching"—the Power of a Pause

Patience-stretching is superfun, supereasy, superuseful . . . and you can start it as early as twelve months. Practice it five times a day and you'll quickly boost your child's ability to be patient . . . which will immediately help reduce bedtime struggles. (*Patience-stretching* is also the key ingredient in the simple *no-cry* sleep-training technique—*twinkle interruptus*—you'll learn on page 254.)

To teach *patience-stretching,* first you must wait until your tot wants something from you.

Next you:

- **Almost give it to him . . . then *stop*! That means you should barely begin to hand him what he's asking for, then suddenly pull it back, raise a finger in the air, and announce "Uh-oh! One second! One second!"** (as if you suddenly remembered you need to do something important).

- **Briefly turn away. Pretend you are busy looking for something for a few seconds.**

- **Finally, give the "payoff." Turn back and cheerily say, "Good waiting! Good waiting!" and give him the thing he wants.**

After a couple of practice runs, start stretching his patience more and more by having him wait a tiny bit longer every few days. In less than a week, he'll easily be able to wait thirty to sixty seconds.

(Amazingly, little kids don't mind waiting—as long as they're confident that we're just about to give them the thing they want.)

If your child has trouble waiting even these few seconds, turn back toward him and use a little *Toddler-ese* to let him know you see how hard it is for him. Say, "I wish we could do that right *now*!!" or "Wait, wait . . . yuck! I wish we just could play *all* day and *never* have to wait!!" Then suggest some things for him to do while he waits and then briefly turn away again.

Step 4: "Magic Breathing"—Nature's Built-In Soother

For many adults, getting calm means eating, sleeping, watching TV, or getting high. Yet within each one of us is an extraordinary, natural stress reducer: deep breathing. Even little kids—starting at eighteen to twenty-four months—can calm their bodies and minds once they learn *magic breathing*.

Here's how.

First, *you* learn. Put your hands together in front of your chest—like you're praying. As you breathe in, swing your hands up and out just in front of your ears . . . and then as you breathe out, let them slowly return to your chest. Repeat the cycle a few times. (You'll look like you're conducting an orchestra.) Do this near your child, so she can watch you practice.

After several demonstrations, your child will eventually want to imitate you. Start with just one or two deep breaths right before eating, napping, roughhousing, or going out to play. (For some extra fun, designate a "magic" spot at home—with special cushions and pictures.)

Don't be pushy. If your little one resists, suggest doing something nice after her *magic breathing*. If she still refuses, say, "No problem." Do a few breaths yourself—you can also sit a stuffed animal next to you and pretend he is doing it with you! Gently encourage her to breathe with you again later that day and the next. If she continues to refuse, keep demonstrating it once or twice a day, but wait a few weeks before asking her to join you again.

Like every other skill, the more your child practices this, the better she'll get . . . and the easier it is for her to switch off her excitement and be quiet in church or at a movie or get ready for bed.

Step 5: Incentives Toddlers Love—"Gossiping," Hand Checks, and Star Charts

Small gifts can grease the wheels of cooperation. Some parents think, *Children should obey simply out of respect.* That's certainly the goal for a six- to eight-year-old, but your three-year-old may need a little extra incentive to cooperate.

(Note: Incentives are not the same as bribery. Bribes are given to encourage *bad* behavior, while incentives are given to encourage *good* behavior.)

A few *Happiest Toddler* techniques boost cooperation and reverse resistance before it even occurs. My favorites are *gossiping,* hand checks, and using star charts.

Gossiping means saying something in a "loud whisper"—pretending you are telling a secret—but letting your tyke overhear you.

For example, a few minutes after thanking your child for his help, cup your hand alongside your mouth and whisper to someone else (even to a doll or a birdie outside), "Psst . . . hey, Mr. Birdie! Steven picked up all his toys . . . really fast!"

Later on, whisper to someone else the same compliment about your child. Your little buddy will think, *Wow, this* must *be true, because I'm hearing it a lot lately.*

Most of us hate being lectured to, yet we're supercurious about things we overhear and we are much more likely to believe them. That's why *gossiping* instantly makes your praise much more effective (and your criticisms, too).

I think of *gossiping* as a "side door" technique, because like storytelling or role-playing (other similar techniques I'll mention later), it teaches a child *indirectly*—through the side door—rather than directly through lectures and explanations.

Hand checks (or hand stamps) are little rewards for when your tot does something you particularly like. Without too much fanfare or cheering draw a check on the back of her hand with a pen or stamp it with a rubber stamp and an ink pad. The idea is to give her this little mark every time you *catch her being good!*

Boost the value of these small checks by taking a few minutes—when she's in bed—to count how many checks she got that day and to remember each good thing she did to earn them (you might also talk about what she might do the next day to earn a check).

Star charts are a more formal way of boosting good behavior (for kids over two).

- Pick three behaviors you want to encourage. Two should be things your child already does (like washing hands or putting on socks) and one should be a little challenge (like eating a bit of broccoli or brushing teeth).

- Have a family meeting. Get together and say, "You do so many really great things! But there are a few things that are kind of hard. Mommy has a fun idea for how to help you do them better."

- Describe what you want him to do.

- Ask his opinion of the best way to keep track of all the good things he does. "Should Mommy put stickers or stars on a chart or poker chips you can keep in your pocket?"

- Decide *together* on a good reward. "Once you get ten stars, should you get a trip to the park? An ice-cream cone? A special gift from the 99-cent store?"

- Make the chart *together*. Decorate it with fun pictures you cut out of magazines.

- Go to the store *together so he can* pick out the stars or stickers he likes the best. (It's superimportant to involve your child in this process . . . after all, it's *his* chart!)

- Hang the chart in a very visible place and let him place the star on it each time he accomplishes his task.

- Every couple of weeks, have another meeting to compliment him on his progress and to change the behaviors he's working on. That keeps the chart interesting. (You can find more tips for successful star charts and family meetings in the book *The Happiest Toddler on the Block*.)

Star charts are fun for toddlers. Your child will get a big scoop of "visual praise" every time he walks by and sees the "big boy" stars prominently displayed. The chart will be even more effective if you let him overhear you *gossip* about his hard work to his stuffed animals.

Step 6: "Playing the Boob"—Boost Cooperation . . . in a Day

We all know how tough it is to raise a toddler—but did you ever stop to think about how tough it is to *be* a toddler?

Your "big boy" may go through the house roaring like a lion, showing off his muscles and stubbornly refusing to give in. But his bravado is often just a cover for his new realization that he's really just a little kid in a big, big world.

Between two and three years of age, your tyke will get really good at comparing things . . . including comparing himself with everyone else. And what he'll realize is that he's weaker, shorter, less eloquent, and slower than everyone but infants (which is why he'll hate being called "a baby"!).

You can't protect your child from every defeat and insecurity. (And you wouldn't want to. It builds character!) But you certainly can boost his confidence and resilience. Of all the *Happiest Toddler* tricks that do this, my favorite is *playing the boob*.

The goofy-sounding idea is for you to act like a boob so your child feels like a winner by comparison. For instance:

- **Act scared when your child growls like a lion.**
- **Have a race. Pretend to make a big effort, but let her win.**
- **Have a pillow fight and let her knock you down with every swipe.**

When you pretend to be a klutz ten times a day, your tot will laugh and feel smart and superior. *Playing the boob* convinces her that you're so "lame" you should be helped, not resisted. Even the most defiant kids usually take pity on us if we occasionally seem like total incompetents.

With these six tricks—the *Fast-Food Rule*, *Toddler-ese*, *patience-stretching*, *magic breathing*, *gossip/hand checks incentives,* and *playing the boob*—you'll prepare your tot for great sleep by building her patience and cooperation.

And now that you have all these tools, it's time to prepare you to tackle sleep problems . . . by busting the myths that get in the way of helping kids sleep successfully.

Don't Believe It! Common Myths About Toddler Sleep

Grandparents, neighbors, and friends are full of advice. Of course they're all very well-meaning, but sometimes they're just flat-out wrong! Here are some of the most common myths you may hear from them.

MYTH 1: *It's normal for little kids to sleep alone.*

FACT: Who really wants to sleep alone? In most cultures, young children sleep with their siblings or parents for years.

Parents are often surprised to learn that bed-sharing increases with age! At three years, 22 percent of kids are doing it; and at four years, 38 percent bed-share at least once a week. Even 10–15 percent of preschoolers still routinely bed-share.

MYTH 2: *Toddlers sleep all night.*

FACT: Actually, video studies show that toddlers wake up from light sleep several times a night. But most of us never know this because our kids usually put themselves back to sleep without a peep.

MYTH 3: *Toddlers need less sleep than infants.*

FACT: Although your toddler's *daytime* sleep will steadily lessen as he gives up his two naps a day, he'll still need eleven to twelve hours of *nighttime* sleep until he reaches five years. And, between four and twelve years of age, his night sleep will barely drop from eleven hours a day to ten.

MYTH 4: *Toddlers should give up their pacifiers, especially at night.*

Fact: It's normal and very comforting to toddlers to suck. In most basic cultures, kids still suckle at the breast until they're three or four years old. Pacifiers can promote a child's confidence and ability to self-soothe in the middle of the night.

Furthermore, many toddlers have a strong genetic tendency to suck. And it's definitely preferable for them to suck a pacifier rather than to get into the habit of thumb sucking, which is much more likely to cause long-term orthodontic problems.

MYTH 5: *A toddler's sleep has nothing to do with his ability to learn or his health.*

FACT: In addition to triggering a host of daytime behavior problems like tantrums, crankiness, aggression, impulsivity, and defiance, sleep deprivation results in "three strikes" against learning: poor attention, poor knowledge acquisition, and poor memory.

Studies have also shown an association in little kids between too little sleep and health issues years later. Surprisingly, a reduction of just one hour of sleep a night during early childhood can affect school-age learning!

For example, Canadian researchers reported that getting less than ten hours of sleep made tots and preschoolers twice as likely to be overweight, have hyperactivity, and do poorly on a cognitive test later in childhood.

It appears that there's a critical period in the early years when inadequate sleep undermines development, even if sleep habits improve later on.

MYTH 6: *Kids naturally fall asleep when they're tired.*

FACT: While most of us (little kids included) fall asleep when we get exhausted, some toddlers actually get *more awake*! They become giddy and start running in circles. In fact, these tots can look like kids with attention-deficit/hyperactivity disorder (ADHD).

And this problem can escalate: *the more tired they get, the harder it is for them to fall asleep, and the more times they wake up during the night.*

MYTH 7: *A night-light can hurt your baby's vision.*

FACT: Nope! Generations of parents have used dim night-lights (four watts) in their infants' bedrooms. Night-lights let us make a quick assessment of our child's well-being without needing to turn on a bright flashlight or room light. Plus, many babies feel safer if they can see familiar surroundings when they wake at 2 A.M. . . . not just a gulf of darkness.

But a 1999 study from Children's Hospital of Philadelphia scared many parents into switching the night-lights off. Researchers said 34 percent of children who used a night-light later became nearsighted.

Fortunately, in the next year, two new studies debunked this claim. Ohio scientists found that only 16.8 percent of the children in their study exposed to night-lights for the first two years became nearsighted, compared with 20 percent of children who slept in darkness. Boston scientists also confirmed there was absolutely no association between night-lights and vision problems.

MYTH 8: *Putting a TV in your tot's room can make bedtime better.*

FACT: *TVs are a huge problem!* Nearly a third of preschoolers have a TV in their room. (And 20 percent of infants do . . . yikes!) In addition, nearly a fifth of parents use the TV or DVD as part of their children's bedtime routine. But using this *electronic pacifier* at night is a bad idea.

Kids with a TV in the bedroom:

- **Watch more TV (that means more violent programming and junk food commercials)**
- **Go to bed twenty to thirty minutes *later***

- Resist sleep (they're twice as likely to fall asleep after 10:00 P.M.)

- Sleep less (they're twice as likely to have trouble waking up in the morning)

- Exercise less

- Have more psychological stress (and perhaps more nightmares)

- Have a higher risk of becoming overweight and obese!

- Can get seriously injured by pulling the TV set on top of themselves

Now, I am not a total puritan about the *boob tube*. It can be a real help as a short-term babysitter . . . and sometimes we all need that. But use TV sparingly (picking gentle shows like *Sesame Street* and nature videos), and turn it off well before bedtime. Better yet, save TV time for special occasions . . . like weekend mornings when it will be a special treat for your little bub, and it may let you snooze an extra thirty minutes.

With these myths vanquished, let's look at what's *true* about toddler sleep.

Normal Sleep for Toddlers

As your child passes her first birthday, sleep continues to be *the* primary brain activity. By two years of age, the average child has spent ninety-five hundred hours (about thirteen months) of her life asleep versus eight thousand hours awake. Between two and five years of age, the amounts of sleep and awake time become about the same.

From one to five years of age, kids sleep twelve to fourteen hours a day, counting naps and nights. (You can expect your two-year-old to nap about two hours a day and your three-year-old to nap one hour a day.)

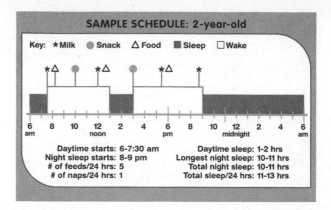

In a worrying trend, toddler sleep has dropped by thirty to forty minutes per night over recent years. It appears that morning wake time has stayed the same, but bedtime has shifted later and later. Most toddlers wake around 7:30 A.M. and go to bed around 9 P.M. (give or take thirty minutes).

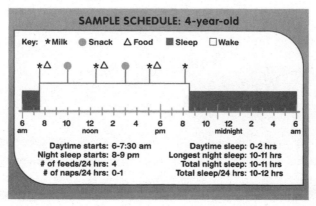

According to the 2004 Sleep in America poll, almost half of toddlers and one-third of preschoolers call out for help some nights (5–10 percent do it more than once a night). Most parents (about 60 percent) return to the bedroom to give reassurance . . . usually staying fifteen minutes until their little sweetie is back asleep. And it usually takes parents at least another fifteen minutes to turn off their minds and fall back to sleep.

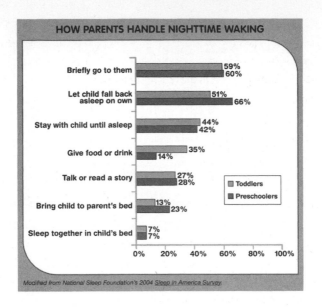

HOW PARENTS HANDLE NIGHTTIME WAKING

- Briefly go to them: 59% / 60%
- Let child fall back asleep on own: 51% / 66%
- Stay with child until asleep: 44% / 42%
- Give food or drink: 35% / 14%
- Talk or read a story: 27% / 28%
- Bring child to parent's bed: 13% / 23%
- Sleep together in child's bed: 7% / 7%

Legend: ☐ Toddlers ■ Preschoolers

Modified from National Sleep Foundation's 2004 Sleep in America Survey.

Fat Chance:
Weighing in on a Serious Issue

Obesity is epidemic today!

It ruins our health, predisposing us to a withering list of serious ailments (including diabetes, heart attacks, cancer, back and hip degeneration, and depression). And it's increasingly clear that weight problems start early—perhaps even in infancy.

In a study of over a thousand children, Canadian researchers found that 26 percent of tots and preschoolers with short sleep (under ten hours a night) became overweight or obese . . . later in childhood (versus 15 percent of kids sleeping ten hours and 10 percent sleeping over eleven hours). In other words, they had two to three times the risk!

And a similar finding was reported by a joint UCLA and University of Washington study as well as a meta-analysis (review of scientific studies) on child sleep and obesity by doctors at Johns Hopkins.

Moreover, kids who are overtired:

- Exercise less (because they're tired)
- Crave more sugar, fat, and empty calories
- Eat more impulsively, even when they're not hungry
- Gain weight from exhaustion-induced metabolic imbalances (insulin resistance, reduced leptin, etc.)

And exhaustion and obesity can become a vicious cycle. As kids gain weight, their necks get fatter. That makes them snore and wake more often, which makes them even more tired!

But the good news is that you have a great opportunity to save your child from a lifetime of struggling with weight if you act now. Here's a bunch of things you can do:

- Eat less food that comes in a box or from a restaurant. (This food is high in fat, sugar, and salt.)
- Eat more fruits, vegetables, beans, and whole grains.
- Aim to have your child get at least ten and a half hours of sleep each night! Avoid sweet drinks. (Juice has as much sugar as soda!)
- Reduce TV time (turn it off during family meals).
- Get outside. Visit the park for some exercise as often as you can.
- Eat dinner as a family at least five times a week. (A great book filled with tips for having fun at the dinner table is *The Family Dinner,* by Laurie David.)

Time for the Big Boy (Girl) Bed?

Fifteen-month-old Will climbed out of his crib while his mom,
Sue, was doing sleep training. "He was okay," she said, "but
I got completely spooked because I suddenly heard his crying
getting closer and closer!"

Your choice when it comes to your little bug's bedtime spot will have a lot to do with her new physical skills.

It's fun to watch her go from standing to walking to running . . . but it's not so much fun when she starts vaulting—commando-style—over the railing. So you'll want to make the transition to the bed before she masters the art of crib escape.

Saying good-bye to your child's crib is a big milestone, but a bittersweet one. (Some parents just can't bear letting go, and they keep this precious souvenir of their baby's early days around long past high school!) Over 90 percent of eighteen-month-olds sleep in a crib, but that gradually drops to about 80 percent at two years and 40 percent by three years of age (see graph below).

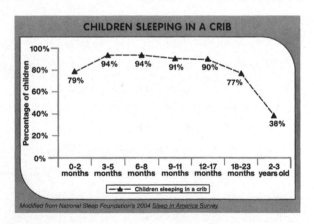

Modified from National Sleep Foundation's 2004 *Sleep in America Survey.*

Since you never know what night your intrepid tot will make that first crib escape, after the first birthday it's wise to put the mattress all the way down and make sure he doesn't have toys or bumpers to climb on. The top of the crib rail should be above his collarbones. And always have a soft rug or carpeting on the floor of the room (with a nonslip undermat), because falls from that height can result in serious injuries.

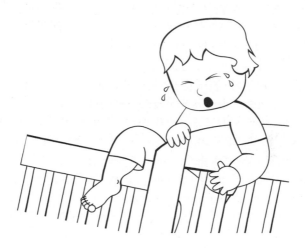

When you're ready to make the switch, remember that tired, cranky toddlers are especially rigid and hate change. So get your child used to the new bed by making it a routine place for quiet play or massage and napping during the day, times when she'll be more flexible.

Your tot will have an easier time with the transition when you continue other familiar sleep cues (like loveys, white noise, your bedtime routine, lullabies, and lavender).

To boost her enthusiasm about the switch:

- Make up little stories or read books about sleeping in bed.

- *Gossip* during the day about what a good job she's doing.

- Take her shopping to pick out special sheets.

- Make a *Beddy-Bye* book that you can peruse together every day with pictures of family members (and your dog!) asleep in their beds. (More about *Beddy-Bye* books on page 240.)

If you're pregnant, it's usually best to move your toddler out of the crib a few months before the baby arrives (assuming your first child is old enough to be out of the crib). If it is already after the birth, you might keep your tot in the crib a while longer. But beware: if you move your toddler to a bed and the next week move the baby into her old crib, your tot may feel jealous—like you gave her beloved possession to the new intruder!

Once in a bed, your toddler can pop out anytime she wants. So you need to (1) childproof the room really well (including electric outlets, curtain cords, and sharp corners), and (2) keep her from roaming outside the room at night.

Use a gate to keep her in her room. If she climbs over it, you may need to spend a little time training her to stay in the room or even close the door. Say something like, "Honey, this is Mr. Gate! Mr. Gate will help you stay in the room . . . so at bedtime after we sing and read and say night-night . . . then we'll close Mr. Gate . . . and he will help you stay safe and happy in your room all night."

If your little gymnast climbs over the gate, you may need to close the door and put a doorknob cover on the inside of the door to her room.

Think Safety First—Especially Now!

Being tired makes kids wired, and this wildness can easily lead to accidents. Just as a tired juggler starts dropping things, tired tots get impulsive and klutzy and prone to all sorts of mishaps.

For preschoolers, the most common bed-related accidents (other than falling out of the crib, which I talked about earlier) result from jumping on the bed or falling out of a bunk bed. I know it's hard to enforce the "no more monkeys jumping on the bed" rule . . . but how crazy do you have to be to let a four-year-old sleep in a top bunk bed? If you know of any parents who let their tots do this, tell them that there are more than thirty-five thousand ER visits each year linked to bunk bed falls . . . with most of them happening to kids between three and five! Worse still, these tend to be head injuries.

That's why the Consumer Product Safety Commission recommends that:

- Children younger than six years old never sleep in the upper bunk.
- Parents use night-lights to help kids see where they're going when they climb down from a top bunk.
- Kids not be allowed to play on upper bunk beds.
- Parents avoid placing bunk beds close to ceiling fans or other ceiling fixtures.

Also, make sure there are no slats or posts in your child's bed where he can catch his head. And finally—I know I've said this before, but I'm a baby doctor, so I have to keep saying it—always have working smoke alarms, fire extinguishers, and an escape plan in case of fire.

If you follow these simple rules, your little monkey should sleep safely and soundly . . . and that will make it much easier for *you* to snooze happily, too.

Keeping Track—How Is Your Tot Actually Sleeping?

I talked about wake/sleep diaries in an earlier section—but here's a quick update in case you skipped that section.

Before you do anything to change your child's sleep, keep a diary for a week or so to get a clear idea of his sleep pattern. (When you're tired, it's easy to forget exactly what was happening a week ago.)

Jot down notes about your little guy's daytime and nighttime behavior:

- **When does he wake up each morning?**
- **How frequent and severe are his outbursts during the day?**
- **When does he take naps? For how long?**
- **In the evening, does he become clingy? Fearful? Hyper?**
- **What time is bedtime—and when do you start and end your bedtime routine?**
- **Is bedtime easy or a struggle?**
- **How long after putting him to bed are you out of the room?**
- **Do you wait until he's asleep?**
- **Does he have trouble settling down? If so, what do you do, and how does it work?**
- **Does he wake up and cry out during the night? If so, when— and for how long?**
- **What do you do in response? Does it help?**

And as long as you're doing this, mark down the other big events of the day, like playdates, school, meals, and poops. There's a sample diary in the appendix to make this job easy.

This type of diary helps you figure out what's going on, what needs to be done, and what progress you're making in resolving sleep issues. This will be a big help as you start using the techniques from the next two chapters.

Crib Notes:
Reviewing the *Happiest Toddler* Way

■ Your little guy is learning some pretty impressive skills (walking, running, speaking . . . arguing!), but in many ways he's still a bit primitive—more *cave-kid* than college student!

■ *SPECIAL TIME:* Special time is a bite-sized bit of your undivided attention. Kids *love* this fun routine!

■ THE *FAST-FOOD RULE:* You'll have a *much* easier time getting your tot to see *your* side if you first show her that you see things from *her* side (even if you don't agree with her).

■ SPEAKING *TODDLER-ESE:* Your child's left brain (the center of language and patience) shuts down when she's upset. *Toddler-ese* is a simple way of talking that tot's understand, even when they "go ape!"

■ *PATIENCE-STRETCHING:* A supereasy way to help your impulsive little friend learn to wait—happily!

■ *MAGIC BREATHING:* Deep-breathing reduces the stress in tots and preschoolers and teaches them self-control.

■ *GOSSIPING:* Supersize the impact of your praise (or criticism) by letting your child overhear you whispering it to someone else.

■ *HAND CHECKS* AND *STAR CHARTS:* These simple cooperation-building steps are key to many of the sleep strategies you're about to learn.

■ *PLAYING THE BOOB:* This is a crazy, fun way to boost cooperation by making your child feel strong and smart—by making yourself seem silly, slow, and weak. Do it ten times a day and your little buddy will become more cooperative . . . before the week is out!

## CHAPTER ELEVEN

Helping Your Little Whirlwind Wind Down for Sleep: One to Five Years

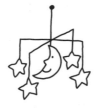

KEY POINTS:

★ Overexcitement, discomfort, stubbornness, poor sleep cues, and the wrong bedtime can lead to troubles at tuck-in time.

★ Make bedtime easier by using *Happiest Toddler* techniques like *Toddler-ese, patience-stretching, playing the boob,* and *gossiping* to build your tot's patience and cooperation—*during the day.*

★ Reduce bedtime struggles by making your child's very own *Beddy-Bye* book—with pictures of every step of his bedtime routine—that you read together during the day.

- ★ Start preparing for bedtime *an hour before* the routine actually starts.

- ★ New routines—from a sleepy-time song to *bedtime sweet talk*—will have your tot loving bedtime in no time.

- ★ You can help your child learn how to *give a little to get a little* by using fair compromises and creative incentives.

- ★ If your tot refuses to stay tucked in, try *twinkle interruptus*—my favorite *no-cry* way of sleep training.

- ★ If all else fails, you can use another sleep-training approach: putting demands "on hold," *pick up/put down,* or the old *cry it out* approach, *longer-and-longer.*

You can learn many things from children. How much patience you have, for instance.

—FRANKLIN P. JONES

Tears and Tantrums: Why Does Your Tot Fight Sleep?

When things are going well, nighttime tuck-ins are a pure pleasure—but when they're not, it's natural to start to fear seeing the sun go down.

Running after your little wild child, wrestling her into PJs, shutting the bedroom door while she's shrieking on the other side— Urrgh!

Many of our little Energizer Bunny toddlers resist bedtime. They hate leaving the thrill of running, climbing, and touching. Around eighteen months they start to go through a very independent phase, where "No!" is their favorite word. And the tired-er they get, the more rigid, hyper, and irritable they become.

In fact, the 2004 Sleep in America poll reported that a third of toddlers—*and half of preschoolers*—regularly stall at bedtime . . . and many downright fight it.

Besides this normal defiance, there are a few other common reasons why your little guy may fight lights-out:

- **He's overexcited—too wound up by TV, roughhousing, or something he's consuming (like sugary juice, sweet snacks, artificial colors and flavors, cold medicine, or a dose of caffeine from colas, Dr Pepper, Mountain Dew, iced tea, or chocolate).**

- **Something is bugging him—bright lights, loud noises, or discomfort (he's teething, too hot, too cold, has a stuffy nose or itchy PJs, ate dinner too late, etc.).**

- **He's nosy and stubborn—doesn't want to go to his room because he wants to see what everyone else is doing.**

- **He's hooked on your help—hasn't yet learned how to fall asleep without you rocking, feeding, and holding him.**

- **He's going through a fearful stage—having difficulty being alone and dealing with a smorgasbord of worries from strangers to dogs to thunder.**

- **Your bedtime timing is off—you're putting him to bed too early (he's not tired) or too late (he's overtired and wired).**

But no matter what the reason, there are lots of ways to help him get past these sleep speed bumps. And one of the best ways is to work on bedtime skills—*all day long.*

Bedtime Routines . . . Toddler Style

There's no doubt about it: a well-planned bedtime routine is the key to great sleep. But good bedtime routines don't just happen. They take a bit of planning, and that planning actually begins . . . *early in the day.*

Step 1—Set Your Tot Up for Nighttime Success . . . During the Day

It should be no surprise that the top cause of bedtime battles is the normal tendency of toddlers to push the limits, especially if they have a spirited and stubborn temperament. And little kids can be extraprimitive (defiant, rigid, and contrary) when they get overly tired at the end of the day. (And of course, *we* get more grumpy and impatient then, too!)

That's why bedtime is the *worst* time to deal with resistance . . . and why *daytime is the best*.

For starters, you'll want to do all the obvious things to keep her healthy and active:

- **Give her lots of sunlight, fresh air, and outdoor play.**
- **Feed her a healthy diet (no caffeine, less sugar, avoid artificial colors and flavors, and include plenty of fiber to avoid constipation!).**
- **Make sure she's napping well, but not so much that it keeps her from being tired at bedtime.**

In addition, your goal is to build such a good relationship during the day that your child naturally wants to cooperate at night. So throughout the day, you'll want to use all the *Happiest Toddler* tricks I discussed in the last chapter—plus a few more—to:

- **Help her feel like a winner.**
- **Stretch her patience.**
- **Make her a bedtime expert through side-door lessons and a Beddy-Bye book.**

Help Her Feel Like a Winner

As I mentioned, our little friends often feel like nonstop *losers!* They're weaker, slower, and can't reach as high or speak as well as everyone else.

That's why your tot will love to stomp in puddles and make a big splash, or say "Boo!" and have you pretend to be frightened. And it's another reason why she may fight you over and over when you're setting a limit . . . she just wants to win a few!

Now, the beautiful thing is that when you *play the boob* with her ten times a day (as recommended in the last chapter), you'll help her feel strong, fast, and smart . . . she will *automatically* become more cooperative. In just days!

In addition, throughout the day I recommend you:

- **Use the *Fast-Food Rule* and *Toddler-ese* whenever she's even a little upset to let her know you understand and respect how she feels—even if you disagree (see pages 211 and 212).**

- **Comment on the good things she does. (*Warning:* It's best to understate praise, not hype it up. For instance, rather than cheering, casually say, "Hmmm . . . you picked up your toys pretty fast today.")**

- **Boost the benefit of this positive attention by *gossiping* about the things you like and using *hand checks* or *star charts* to show your appreciation (see page 215).**

- **Give her options ("I know you're having fun, but we really have to leave. Do you want to stay for two more minutes or leave right now?").**

Stretch Her Patience

When you practice *patience-stretching* five times a day and also do a few *magic breaths* you will help your little cave-kid master the skills of patience and self-restraint, which will naturally help her to wind down faster at bedtime.

Make Her a Bedtime Expert

Children hate sermons. They're much more likely to do what they see than to do what they're told. So skip the lecture, and instead, teach your tot important lessons—through the *side door*.

I mentioned this concept earlier, but I'd like to explain it a little more because I think it is such a help for parenting young children. We all stand guard at the "front door" of our minds, rejecting messages that seem bossy . . . and even rejecting praise that seems excessive or insincere! Yet all of us (kids and grown-ups) are very trusting of what we *overhear*—in other words, information entering the "side door" of our minds.

Here are three fun ways to sneak through your tyke's "side door" to plant suggestions of kindness and cooperation without her feeling pushed into it: *gossiping*, doll play, and fairy tales.

Gossiping (described on page 215) means letting your child overhear you commenting to someone about things she's doing that you want to encourage (or discourage).

Your child is overhearing you talk to others *all the time,* so use those opportunities to give little messages that will boost the behaviors you like and reduce ones you don't. If you *gossip* your little bits of praise or criticism five or ten times a day, you'll see definite changes within the week!

Say things like:

"Psst, Daddy, Rosie came to cuddle with me for naptime just three seconds after I called her! That was superfast! She's getting to be such a big girl."

"Psst, hey, Grandma, Marnie kissed her dollies, then cuddled her teddy and did two big magic breaths, and then she had really sweet dreams."

Another way to pass side-door messages to your munchkin is through *doll play*.

Doll (or puppet) play is silly and fun, and little kids are often more open to advice from a little doll than from Mama!

When two-year-old Sadie balked at the sight of her toothbrush, her dad, Jonah, turned to her Buzz Lightyear doll and said, "Hold on . . . I need to check with Buzz on this."

Then Jonah "whispered" to Buzz, loud enough for Sadie to overhear: "Buzz, Sadie needs your help! She doesn't want to brush her teeth, but I don't want the bad sugar bugs to make holes in them. What do you think?"

Jonah put his ear next to Buzz's helmet and pretended to listen. "What's that, Buzz? You want Sadie to have happy teeth and get rid of the bugs? And you'll be very proud of her if she brushes? That's great! And can I give her a hand check for doing a good job? Thanks, Buzz!"

Sadie brushed her teeth, keeping one eye on Buzz the whole time. Then Jonah gave her a hug and a hand check and "gossiped" with Buzz about what a great little girl she was.

Your tot will love switching roles during doll play. For instance, you or she can be the voice of the Baby Bear ("Waaa, waaa, I don't want to go to bed yet!") and then she can switch and be the voice of the Mama Bear ("Okay, let's play for two more minutes. Then you have to brush away the sugar bugs on your teeth, okay?").

Another way to sneak messages through the side door is with your own fairy tales—made-up stories with hidden lessons. Kids love listening to fairy tales—over and over again—which lets their hidden messages slowly sink in, without nagging or threats.

So cuddle up with your angel sometime during the day and tell a tale in which Billie the Bunny (it's best to use animal characters, not people) struggles to get his PJs on fast so he has time to read some fun books, or go to bed early so he can have really fun dreams of being a superhero!

And to keep it fun, feel free to add a couple of silly details to your stories to make them more memorable. "And then she brushed her teeth . . . and she kissed her pet worm good night!"

(You can read lots more about fairy tales and other great side-door tips and tricks in the book *The Happiest Toddler on the Block*.)

Create a Beddy-Bye Book!

Another trick that works miracles at reducing bedtime resistance is sitting with your tot and reading together his personal *Beddy-Bye* book, every day.

Here's how to make one.

Take your little buddy to the store to buy stickers that he likes, colored construction paper, a hole punch, and a nice loose-leaf binder (so you can add and remove pages at will). Then at home, you and your buddy can work together to decorate the covers of your new book.

Inside the book, on the first and last pages, make a happy face and write, "The 4 Rules of Happy Sleep." Feel free to make up your own rules, but here are some good ones:

- **Happy, clean hands.**
- **Brush, brush sugar bugs off your teeth.**
- **PJs feel good!**
- **I'm snug as a bug in bed.**

Over the next few days, take some photos: you buying special sheets; your tot's star chart; eating dinner; playing before bedtime (lights dimmed); putting on PJs; brushing teeth; turning on the white noise; doing *bedtime sweet talk*; prayers; kisses from Mommy and Daddy; lights-out; your tyke sleeping; waking up happy with the birds.

Also, take shots of other family members (including pets) getting ready for bed and sleeping. And while you're at it, include more fun sleep pictures from magazines and even scribbles your toddler made about happy dreams.

Under each photo or drawing, add little captions, like:

- "Maya, brushing away the sugar bugs"
- "Daddy and Theo reading fun stories . . . that feels good!"
- "Twyla's eyes are getting comfy and closing"

Finally, put in a few special nature pictures . . . perhaps a sunny sky and the moonlit night, or some animals sleeping.

Read it together during the day and ask, "And what comes next?" so he's totally in sync with the routine. And from time to time during the day, ask him out of the blue if he can help you remember all four of the rules. Looking at his book every day will quickly help your little cutie become more cooperative at night.

Your *Beddy-Bye* book will become another great treasure from your child's early years!

Step 2—Develop a Great Bedtime Routine

If you don't already have a sleepy-time routine in place, now's the time to create one. Here's what to do.

The Prebed Routine (30–60 Minutes)

As the evening is drawing to a close, give your tot a few signals that bedtime is approaching:

- **Dim the lights in the house.**
- **Do quiet play (not roughhousing).**
- **Turn off the TV.**
- **Put on white noise in the background.**
- **If you think your child has teething pain, ask your doctor if some medicine might help.**

The "Get in Bed" Routine (20–30 Minutes)

Each family picks a slightly different bedtime routine. The key is to make your routine pleasant, loving, calming, and consistent.

As I mentioned in an earlier chapter, Philadelphia researchers found that parents who started a three-step bedtime routine (bath, massage, and quiet cuddling or singing a lullaby) saw success within two weeks. Their children (seven to thirty-six months old) fell asleep faster . . . and slept longer!

And, as an extra bonus, the toddlers were less likely to call out to their parents or get out of their crib or bed.

Besides baths and massage, here are other routines many parents opt for.

When it's time to start your routine, don't invite resistance by asking, "Are you ready for bed?" Rather, start with an enthusiastic "Okay, all kids! Time for bed!" Make a hand sign for "bedtime" and begin a countdown before you start to sing a *sleepy-time song*. (Just make up a little ditty with words like, "It's sleepy-time!" or "Time to go to bed!"—perhaps to a familiar tune like "Happy Birthday.")

As you sing, make a simple "let's sleep" gesture—perhaps putting your hands together like a pillow and resting your head on them.

Right before you start your bedtime routine, make your princess's room perfect by:

- **Dimming the lights**
- **Keeping it cool (66°F–72°F is best)**
- **Warming the sheets (use a hot water bottle or a little microwavable wheat bag that's removed when you tuck your munchkin in)**
- **Using a pleasant smell (a drop of lavender oil on the mattress or headboard is nice)**
- **Plugging in a small night-light**
- **Putting up a dream catcher or a picture of Mommy and Daddy to "protect" your sweetie all night**

All kids enjoy saying "Good night!" to their toys. Prayers, lullabies, and bedtime stories are wonderful sleep steps, too, and a pacifier or a last sip of water can also help bring on the sandman.

(Offer water or caffeine-free mint or chamomile tea, but avoid cavity-promoting juices or sugary drinks at bedtime. Also limit pre-sleep breast-feeding or sucking on a bottle to about thirty minutes, because milk and formula also create cavity-producing bacteria.)

Loveys like a blankie or a teddy bear are great allies in your bedtime routine. Think of them as stepping-stones to maturity and independence. These faithful friends are called transitional objects because they give kids the courage to take steps away from their mama and daddy and transition away from the family into the great big world.

If your tot doesn't have a favorite lovey, you can pick a soft, cuddly one to carry around with you all day. Within a few weeks, your tot may start to get interested—associating the toy with your sweet cuddling—and a friendship with the lovey may begin.

Make sure your lovey has no bits or buttons attached to it that might cause choking. And make sure you have a spare, just in case the first is lost or needs to be cleaned. Never remove a lovey as punishment. Far from making kids behave better, it can trigger resentment and insecurity.

And don't forget that old familiar sleep cue, white noise.

But, as your toddler's mind gets more active, you may find that softer sounds just don't work and you need a *rougher* white noise, like that on *The Happiest Baby* CD, which includes specially filtered womb or rain sound containing a mix of both shushy high-pitch and rumbly low-pitch frequencies.

White noise is an even better sleep cue than a teddy bear, because it's simple to replace if you lose it, and it's easier to wean later (for white noise weaning tips see page 180).

Other nice ideas for your bedtime routine might include:

- **A warm bath (with the lights dimmed low)**
- **A coconut oil massage (stroke the forehead from the eyebrows up to the scalp, slightly pulling your child's eyes open with each stroke . . . this will make her want to close her eyes)**

- Sprinkling a little "magic dust" around the room (sounds crazy, but it really works)

And last but certainly not least is my favorite *Happiest Toddler* bedtime routine, *bedtime sweet talk*.

The Happiest Toddler Way

BEDTIME SWEET TALK: THE POWER OF POSITIVE THOUGHTS

One of the sweetest rewards of parenting is cuddling with your little munchkin right before he slips into slumber. Gentle rocking, soft massages, and cooing lullabies are perfect ways to give quality love at the end of a long, tiring day.

And another wonderful way to bring the day to a close is with a routine called *bedtime sweet talk*.

The last moments—right before sleep—your child's mind is wide open, like a little sponge soaking up your loving words. *Bedtime sweet talk* takes advantage of that golden opportunity to fill your tyke's sleepy mind with gratitude for all the wonderful things he did that day and to nurture a sense of optimism about all the things he may do and experience tomorrow.

Here's how you can use this routine, with kids as young as one year old:

- Once your tot is tucked in, snuggle up next to him.

- In a soft, understated way recount some of his fun experiences and acts of kindness from the day just past.

- If you gave him any hand checks, count them and see if together you can remember how he earned them.

- Think about the next day and list a few things that might happen and good deeds he may do.

("Tomorrow, I wouldn't be surprised if you climbed all the way to the top of the play structure. And you might even help Teacher Janet pick up all the blocks again!")

The Blessed Binky: You Could Stop It Now, but Do You Really Want To?

Sucking is deeply soothing for little kids, and that's why it's one of the 5 S's. But parents are constantly pushed by others (or by that little voice in their head) to break the binky habit.

If you're feeling that pressure, take a moment . . . for a little reassurance.

First, remember that in traditional cultures, toddlers often suck at the breast until four years of age.

Second, some kids have a strong genetic drive—on one or both sides of the family—to fall in love with a soothing object (binky, thumb, teddy, or security blanket), that's why removing the paci often leads to more thumb sucking. (Pacis are better than thumbs because sucking on fingers can seriously distort the palate and teeth, leading to the need for uncomfortable—and expensive— braces later.)

Third, it may sound silly to say this, but your tyke's pacifier may become one of his deepest, closest friends.

And fourth, nobody ever goes to college using a pacifier.

However, if you're tired of picking up the binky your tot keeps tossing out the crib, or if he's getting ear infections (from the paci), or you're just ready to wean it, here's how to do the job:

- Use *patience-stretching* and *magic breathing* every day to help him learn to calm his worries and delay his desires— without sucking.

- Encourage him to use other loveys like a blankie, teddy, or one of your silky scarves. ("Honey, I'll find your paci in a second. Hold teddy while Mommy is getting it for you.")

- *Gossip* to his stuffed animals about how he went all morning without the paci.

- Tell fairy tales about a bunny who said good-bye to his paci but had a magic teddy that made him feel happy every time he hugged it.

- Limit pacifier use to certain situations like sleep or stressful times when your tot needs calming.

- Establish a couple of "paci-free" times during the day. Start with thirty minutes—after a nap is a good time. I recommend you use a timer so your child doesn't keep bugging you to have it. ("Sweetie, I know you want your binky . . . right now! . . . but we have to wait for Mr. Dinger to ring and tell us you can have it. Remember, that's the rule! Hey, do you want to play with your cars or read a book while we're waiting for that crazy old Mr. Dinger to ring?")

- Don't say you're giving the paci to another baby. That may create jealousy every time he sees a baby with a paci! (One parent told his three-year-old that he was sending it to Santa's workshop to make it into a new playground for little kids!)

- Discuss together when to give the binky away. You might choose a special day, like his birthday (I prefer the fourth).

- Make sure there's something in it for him! Your tot will have an easier time separating from his old friend if he gets something in exchange (like a great big-boy toy that you shop for together!).

- Put fun stickers around the "bye-bye paci, hello (put in the name of the special gift)" day on a calendar. Give him a red pen to cross off each day as you count down to *the* day.

Be positive, but don't get *too* excited. Some kids suddenly balk and decide they're not ready yet. ("Mommy, sometimes I'm not a big boy!") And you don't want to make your child feel like a failure or make him think that he's let you down. ("Okay . . . I guess you love it so much you don't want to say bye-bye to it yet . . . maybe next week?")

Helping Spirited, Resistant Kids Obey the Limits

By the end of the day, many of us start losing our patience. That's why bedtime struggles often make us feel tempted to just grab our little screamers and *make them obey.*

But that's not a great idea.

Giving an ultimatum to your exhausted little cave-kid can paint her into a corner and make her dig in her heels and get even more defiant . . . especially if your child's temperament is naturally tenacious and stubborn—or if she is simply a normal eighteen-month-old stuck in the midst of her *terrible twos!*

Now, I'm not saying you should be a wimp. Sometimes you *must* seize control of the situation and pull your child in from the gutter or make her put down the scissors. But nighttime is the worst time for conflicts: you're both tired, you have to get work done . . . and your primitive little friend has nothing better to do than scream for hours! So smart parents sidestep brute force and try to find more diplomatic solutions.

Once again, you'll be *much* more successful avoiding conflicts at night if you spend a little time boosting cooperation *during the day.* Do this by using the *Happiest Toddler* tools you already know— like *playing the boob, patience-stretching, Beddy-Bye* book, and so on.

Sophia and Russell found they could defuse bedtime struggles with Tessa by playing the boob. They started having nightly races to see who could brush teeth the fastest, get PJs on the fastest, and so on (the winner got a "princess" hand stamp).

But no matter how hard you try, there will inevitably be some struggles you just can't avoid. That's when a new approach can come to the rescue—*win-win* solutions.

Give a Little, Get a Little—the Win-Win Solution (for Kids Over Two)

The best resolution to conflict is where both sides feel like winners!

Imagine that your stubborn little toddler is whining because he doesn't want to get ready for bed. The car game you're playing is just too much fun!

To get things moving, look for a way you *both* can get a good bit of what you want:

1. Sincerely acknowledge his feelings in *Toddler-ese:* "Sammy, you are having sooo much fun! You love, love, l-o-v-e playing with your cars! I wish we could play with them all night!" *or* "I totally get it! You want to play more and you don't even feel tired yet. You say, 'No way, Mom! I'm not ready for bed yet!' "

2. Once he calms, it's your turn to say what *you* want: "But, sweetheart, you know the rule. It's sleepy-time, and all little boys have to put on their PJs and get ready for bed."

3. If he protests, offer a respectful *win-win* compromise: "Okay, you win, you win! I know you really, really, r-e-a-l-l-y want to keep playing, and you did such a great job today—washing your hands and bringing your dish to the sink—so tonight I'll break the rule a tiny bit. You can play for five more minutes— until Mr. Dinger rings and says it's time for us to read stories in bed. All you have to do first is put on this PJ shirt and brush your teeth superfast. Deal?"

4. When you make a deal, look each other in the eye and shake hands on it. And let Mr. Dinger be the bad guy enforcing the deal ("It's not up to me, it's up to Mr. Dinger").

A great way to find a win-win solution with an older toddler or preschooler is through a family meeting (see chapter 10). Here's how two smart parents solved their problem with this approach.

Night after night, two-and-a-half-year-old Asher called his parents back to his room after lights-out. He wanted a drink, a hug, another book. He was an expert at persuasion: "I really, really, really need a kiss from Daddy."

So Matty and Masha decided to have a meeting with Asher during the day. They sat down and talked about all the fun things they did last weekend and all the great things that Asher was doing now that he was a big boy (so much bigger than his little brother, Max). But they all had one problem. Asher didn't like it when he had to go to bed, and they didn't like it when he kept calling them back.

"But I have a good idea," said Masha. "We'll give you two of these poker chips every night at bedtime. We'll still come back whenever you want us to, but the new rule is that each time we come you'll give us one of the poker chips, just like the way we pay for something at the store.

"If you don't need us to come back at all, then you can keep the poker chips, or give them to us and we'll give you a special gift for each poker chip. Should you get a special sticker? Or would you like a little bag of goldfish crackers for two poker chips? What do you think would be a good gift?"

Asher decided he wanted the goldfish crackers. And they all agreed and shook hands on their new deal. That night at bedtime, right before brushing his teeth, Matty played the boob by pretending that he couldn't remember what they'd agreed on.

He asked Asher for help: "I can't exactly remember our deal. We give you two poker chips and then you give us one each time you call for us to come. But in the morning what do we give you for each poker chip? Was it a quarter?" And Asher instantly chimed in, in his cute little lisp, "Goldfiss!!" "Oh right, goldfish crackers. You love them so much!"

About five minutes after lights-out, Asher called out, "I'm thirsty, Mama!" Masha came right away and said, "Hi, sweetheart, I can get you some water or juice, but remember the rule: you have to give me one of your poker chips—or if you're not too-too thirsty you could wait until morning and then get all the water you want for free, okay?"

Asher's face got serious and he looked at his hand (holding the chips) and then at Masha and then at his hand again. Then he said, "That's okay, Mama, I don't need water so much right now." Masha reminded him that she'd be happy to come back again if he got thirsty. And he said, "That's okay, I'll just hug Knuckles [his stuffed dog]." "Okay," Masha said. "Just let me know if you need me later. Night-night . . . don't let the bugs bite!"

Masha said, "By the way he was clutching those chips, I knew I was going to get sleep that night. The next morning he proudly presented the chips to us at the breakfast table. And we exchanged them for his crackers (which he put away in his room for later!).

"The rest of the week, there were only two times he exchanged a poker chip for me to come and cuddle. The next week we had another meeting and changed the incentive: Asher decided that he wanted one chip to get a two-minute piggyback ride and he wanted to keep the goldfish crackers for the two-chip exchange."

As you can see, you should never threaten or criticize your child for not getting the tokens. Just cheerfully remind her that she has a choice. And if she doesn't do the job today, maybe she'll do it tomorrow.

Of course, if your child refuses your deal or breaks her promise, you can try giving her another chance ("Okay, I can see you're not ready yet, so should Mr. Dinger give you one or two more minutes to play before we have to put on PJs and brush teeth?"). But, if she still refuses, you may just have to skip the tooth brushing that night (it's too hard to do with a screaming child anyway). Tell her she leaves you no choice but to pick her up and take her to bed—so she doesn't learn that whining gets her what she wants.

When you combine win-win solutions with all your bedtime sleep cues, you'll solve many sleep problems quickly. Here's a quick review of all the tricks you can use at this stage to get your little cub tucked in happily:

- **Build confidence during the day with *Toddler-ese, patience-stretching, magic breathing, gossiping, playing the boob*, sticker charts, role-playing, fairy tales, and a *Beddy-Bye* book.**

- **Have thirty to sixty minutes of quiet time with the lights dimmed and the TV off before you start your routine. A warm bath and a massage can also relax your child.**

- **Let your sweetie say good night to all the toys!**

- **Use white noise, loveys, storybooks, lullabies, lavender, and *bedtime sweet talk* to help your child drift off. A pacifier is fine at this stage, too.**

- **Offer compromises . . . both during the day and at night . . . so everyone can win.**

Timing Is Everything!—Picking the Right Moment for Bed

Sometimes when we're trying to understand why a child is fighting bedtime, we overlook the obvious: we picked the *wrong* time! If your little one is yelling, "No, no, no!" at nighttime, ask yourself these questions:

Is bedtime *too early*? Look for these clues:

- **Your tot fights falling asleep for thirty to sixty minutes.**
- **She shows no sign of fatigue at bedtime.**
- **She wakes up in the middle of the night or very early the next day, refreshed and ready to go.**

Is bedtime *too late*? Look for these clues:

- **Your child fights falling asleep for thirty to sixty minutes.**
- **She has trouble waking in the morning; she's extra cranky and moody during the day; and she falls asleep during car or stroller rides.**
- **She shows clear signs of fatigue at bedtime (rubbing her eyes, blinking, yawning, getting silly and wild, acting cranky, having accidents).**

If you think bedtime is too early, try pushing the bedtime routine *fifteen minutes later* every two to three nights.

If you think bedtime is too late, start the routine *fifteen minutes earlier* every two to three nights. Either approach should work within a week or two.

Travel and Daylight Savings Time

Rebecca asked for medication to help two-year-old Luke sleep on the long flight from L.A. to South Africa. Her doctor suggested Benadryl, but he neglected to tell her to try a test dose the week before they traveled.

This was a big mistake! Luke was one of the many children who get wired—not sleepy—when they take Benadryl.

*Rebecca said she gave him a spoonful shortly after takeoff
and he cried for two hours straight, until he fell asleep out of
exhaustion. Needless to say, the trip was a nightmare for her,
Luke, and everyone around them.*

Anything that disrupts the circadian rhythm can lead to sleep
problems, including traveling (especially to the east) or moving
the clocks forward in the springtime for daylight savings time.

When you take your tot on short, close trips (under five days and
fewer than three time zones) try to stick to your home time zone
and keep your regular day schedule and bedtime routines.

If you travel farther and longer, jump to the new time zone and
provide your child with lots of morning daylight and exercise
to reset his brain's melatonin release. Offer familiar bedtime
routines (including his all-important *white noise!*), and bring
along his cherished loveys and even his comfy old sheets. Dim
the lights an hour before bedtime, turn off the TV for two or three
nights, and avoid late meals.

Crossing time zones to the east is tougher for us than crossing
time zones traveling west. That's because our natural circadian
clock actually *wants* to be awake twenty-five to twenty-six hours
a day. So it's easy for the brain to absorb an extra hour or two—
but removing a few hours from our day (as when we fly from
L.A. to New York) gives us a bad case of *jet lag,* which can take
several days to recover from.

So if you're planning to travel east across more than three time
zones, move your tot's sleep and wake times a little earlier. Start
a week before, and move things fifteen minutes earlier every day
or two (starting with an earlier wake-up and then shifting all naps
and meals a bit earlier as well).

The key to making a good transition to a new time zone when
traveling to the east is to get plenty of daytime light and avoid
sleeping too much during the day. The first day or two, wake your

child if he's sleeping more than one hour later than his normal waking time. Move his naptime earlier if he is very tired during the day.

Ask your doctor if melatonin or an antihistamine like diphenhydramine (Benadryl) might help your toddler sleep on a long flight. But remember Rebecca's experience with Luke, and make sure you test *any* medicine with your child before you travel!

One way to make daylight savings time a little easier is to make a gradual change in your child's bedtime before the day you actually *spring forward*. Shift dinner and bedtime fifteen minutes earlier a week ahead of time. Then shift it another fifteen minutes three days later, again fifteen minutes earlier on the day of daylight savings, and then again three days later.

Sleep Training—*Twinkle Interruptus, Cry It Out,* and Other Ways to End Bedtime Delays

Toddlers hate going to bed because life is endlessly fun in the living room and—well, let's face it—pretty darn boring in the bedroom!

So some vault over the side of the crib like little commandos and emerge, bleary eyed, into the festival of light and activity just outside their door. Others keep reappearing after lights-out, like an actor taking extra bows at the end of a play, saying "I'm thirsty!" "I'm scared," "I have to pee-pee," "I need *Daddy* to kiss me."

If your little artiste refuses to leave the stage, it's time to get your sleepy-time routine back on track . . . quickly and lovingly. Here's how.

First, remember that nighttime success starts with daytime encouragement. So please review all the steps I described on pages 236–41.

Then, try out one of the following sleep-training tricks. I recommend beginning with my all-time favorite approach, *twinkle interruptus.*

The Happiest Toddler Way

TWINKLE INTERRUPTUS

Bedtime was frustration time for Aaron because two-year-old Emma would make him sing "Twinkle, Twinkle Little Star" over and over for an hour, until she fell asleep.

"She insists that I sing 'Twinkle' to her about ten gazillion times . . . again and again!" he said. "Sometimes she seems to be asleep and I'll try to ease myself off her bed, but if I make any tiny sound, she'll immediately grumble out a half-asleep demand, 'Twinkle!!!' and I know I'll be stuck there for another twenty minutes, until she's fast asleep."

To save Aaron's sanity, I taught him a simple trick based on *patience-stretching*. For a week, I had Aaron do two things to prepare Emma for success:

1. Use a rough, rumbly white noise for all Emma's naps and night sleep. About an hour before bedtime, he quietly played the rain on the roof track from the *Happiest Baby on the Block* CD—and continued it from lights-out until morning, increasing the sound—night by night—until it was as loud as a shower.

2. Practice *patience-stretching* five times a day. Soon Emma was able to wait a whole minute without complaining.

Now Aaron was ready to start the *twinkle interruptus* strategy.

That first night, Aaron put on the white noise, snuggled with Emma, and sang her song for a few minutes. Then he shot his finger up into the air—as if he'd suddenly remembered something important—and announced, "Wait! Wait! I forgot to kiss Mommy. Here, hold teddy. I'll be RIGHT back." He hurried out for five seconds.

Emma's practice with patience-stretching during the week gave her the confidence to wait those few seconds. She remembered that when Daddy said "Wait! Wait!" and left, he would be right back.

Soon Aaron slid back into the room whispering, "Good waiting! Good waiting!" He immediately cuddled up with his little girl and started singing again. After another few minutes, he repeated the same "Wait! Wait!" routine, but this time he disappeared for fifteen seconds.

Again, Emma tolerated it fine, and when he returned, he repeated, "Good waiting! Good waiting!" and sang to her until she fell asleep.

The next night, Aaron repeated the same actions—but his first exit lasted for thirty seconds and his second lasted for a full minute. And when he tiptoed in at the end of the second time, Emma was fast asleep. And she stayed asleep for the night!

You'll really have fun with this approach. It works about 75 percent of the time for kids over eighteen months of age (and I've even had success with *twinkle interruptus* in helping a few twelve-month-olds sleep train without a tear!).

If your tot cries when you leave, immediately return to comfort her—she may be experiencing some special stress, anxiety, or fear. Over the next few days, keep doing *patience-stretching* during the day, white noise for all sleeping times, and make sure she has a lovey to hold when you go away. Next, when you try *twinkle interruptus* again, don't leave the room. After saying, "Wait! Wait!" simply go across the room and pretend to be searching for something. Then return to the bed again and say, "Good waiting!" Gradually increase the amount of time you spend on the other side of the room. If she tolerates that well after a couple of days, try leaving the room for a short period again.

Please don't think of this as *devious*. But everyone is tired and has low frustration tolerance at bedtime, so this is a better time to be a little tricky than to enter into a battle of wills.

Putting Demands "On Hold" (for Kids Over Eighteen Months)

Here's another *no-tears* approach that works with persistent kids. If your tot runs over your rules like a steamroller, try this little *Happiest Toddler* technique (another twist on *patience-stretching*) to put her unreasonable demands "on hold."

First, spend a week practicing *patience-stretching* five times a day and using white noise for all sleep. Once your tot gets used to all this, you're ready to put her unreasonable demands "on hold." Here's how.

When your sleepy tyke toddles up to the night gate in her PJs and pleads for water, come immediately and say, "Okay, sweetheart, Mommy's here, Mommy's here." Listen to her request and say, "Sure, honey, sure." But then raise one finger (as if you just remembered something important) and exclaim, "Wait! Wait! I forgot something! I'll be back . . . really fast!" And tell her to cuddle her lovey until you come back. (She'll be familiar with all this from her experiences with *patience-stretching* during the day.)

Hurry out of view for five seconds. Then, return and innocently ask, "Honey, I'm *so* sorry I forgot—what do you want?" Or say, "Oh darn! Silly Mommy! I forgot the water! I'm sorry, honey. I'll be back in just a sec!" Then leave for ten seconds, but this time actually get it for her.

The next time she summons you, do the "Wait! Wait!" routine again—but this time, disappear for fifteen seconds. When you return, ask what she wants, but then do the routine again and return thirty seconds later with the water.

Over a few days, you can build the waiting period up to one and then two minutes. Eventually, your tot will discover that asking for things has turned into a pretty boring, no-fun game.

(Your little pup may get tired and fall asleep on the floor while she's waiting for your return. So leave a pillow and blanket on the floor by the door gate in case she chooses to fall asleep there instead of in bed.)

If your sweetie gets impatient and starts yelling, wait five seconds, then return and acknowledge her frustration (in your best *Toddler-ese*). Then repeat your "Wait! Wait!" routine and disappear for another fifteen seconds.

Taking It to the Next Level

If these simple approaches don't work, and your tot still demands your presence while she's falling asleep, it might be time to consider a more direct method of sleep training.

Back in chapter 8, I outlined two different approaches called *pick up/put down* and *longer-and-longer* (this is the old Ferber-style graduated extinction, or *cry it out*, method). At the toddler stage, you can add a few twists—like reviewing with your child her *Beddy-Bye* book during the day, doing doll play, and practicing *patience-stretching* and *magic breathing*—but regardless of what you do, you should be prepared for extra friction from your tenacious little cave-kid if you choose to use the *cry it out* method. Here's a look at both methods.

Pick Up/Put Down, Toddler Style

In *pick up/put down* (or fading), play a strong white noise in the room and sit quietly next to the crib or bed, responding to your tot's cries by picking him up and cuddling—but only until he calms.

Stay in the room until he falls deeply asleep. Then, over the course of several days, as he gradually cries less and less, move your chair farther from the crib or bed and closer to the door (see page 191 for more details).

And now you can add *twinkle interruptus* to this routine. Practice *patience-stretching* five times a day for a week. Then at night, once your lovebug seems to be doing better and falling asleep with less picking up, begin saying, "Wait! Wait! Hold your teddy! I'll be right back!" and go to the other side of the room—or leave the room completely—for short periods.

If he's already sleeping in his own bed, make a rule that you'll stay in the room . . . but only if he stays in his bed. If he gets out of bed, have a family meeting with your tot to discuss it (for a description of this, see page 217).

At this meeting, say something like this:

"I know sometimes you want Mommy to come back and be with you after you go to bed, but the rule is that kids, pets, and mommies have to sleep so we can be happy and play the next day!

"So let's make a plan. When I tuck you into bed, I'll give you two special passes. If you call me back to visit you for water or an extra kiss or for a back scratch or to pee-pee, or even for any reason, I'll come fast—but you have to give me one of your special passes.

"But in the morning, if you still have your passes, you can exchange them for a special gift. What would you like? Stars? Special stickers? A shiny new quarter? A cookie?"

"Longer-and-Longer" or Cry It Out (CIO), Toddler Style

Thirteen-month-old Arianna was still getting up every couple of hours at night to breast-feed. Her mom, Dawn, was a working mom, and she worried that she'd get sick or have a car accident or not have enough energy to play with Ari if she kept up this demanding schedule. But she also worried that Ari would feel rejected if she didn't nurse her at night.

Finally, at the insistence of her mom and husband, Dawn started a CIO routine. And she was amazed! "The first night, Ari cried for thirty minutes before falling asleep and then woke up for a feeding five hours later. And the second night, she fell asleep after five minutes of fretting and slept for an incredible eight hours!"

Dawn told me, "Now, she just whimpers at about 1 A.M. and falls back to sleep. I think this has saved my marriage!"

If you're at your wit's end and need help fast, CIO may be appropriate. Before trying it, *be sure to read the section on this technique on page 190.* You'll follow the same procedure at this age, but be aware that toddlers and preschoolers can be tougher to train.

Why? Because they're much more tenacious. They can scream for an hour or more and vomit every time! And once they're out of the crib, they can go right to the door.

To increase your odds of success, use white noise at bedtime for a week beforehand. Then follow this drill.

Once you close the door, let your darling cry for three minutes and then pop your head in just to make sure she's okay and let her see that you haven't deserted the planet. Say, "I love you, sweetie, but it's time to sleep . . . so night-night, sleep tight."

Some parents find that a longer visit works. However, this is more likely to give your child false hope that you'll rescue her and encourage *more* shrieking.

After you close the door again, wait five minutes and repeat step one. After that, wait ten minutes and do it again. Then peek in every fifteen minutes until she falls asleep. If she wakes in the middle of the night, you can do a feeding if you want—but then repeat the same *longer-and-longer* method.

If your tot barfs, come in but *don't say too much*—just make sure she's fine, clean up the mess, and say, "I love you, sweetheart; everything is fine. Night-night," and leave the room.

The first night, stubborn little kids can cry for an hour or more—and the second night, they may go on for even longer (read about *extinction bursts* on page 190). But don't lose your determination. If you give in after an hour of crying and pick your angel up, you'll end up teaching her exactly the wrong lesson: *if you just yell long enough, you'll get what you want.*

So if you can, hold out. Usually the third night is *much* better . . . and by the fourth night, your tot should be falling asleep fast and sleeping through the night.

If things aren't better by the fourth night, step back and think about whether your bedtime is too early or too late; if there's some special stress in her life; or whether you're sending mixed signals by talking to her too much or staying too long when you pop in.

Also, if you have a cautious, sensitive child, think about whether she may need a gentler approach, with more visits and a little patting and reassurance when you enter—or one of the *no-tears* sleep techniques.

If, on the other hand, you have a spirited, tenacious, defiant cave-kid, offering too much attention will just encourage her . . . so make your visits cheerful but brief.

Hang in there!

If you do need to use CIO, try to keep some perspective (and a sense of humor) during this miniordeal. Remember that while these scream-filled evenings seem endless, they'll be over soon—and all of you will be sleeping better in just a few days. So stay focused on your goal, and do some *magic breathing* to help you relax. And keep telling yourself that millions of parents have survived this experience (they're the ones who passed on the classic advice, "put cotton in your ears and gin in your stomach")—and you'll survive it, too!

Crib Notes:
Reviewing *The Happiest Toddler* Way

■ Good bedtime routines start . . . *early in the day*.

■ Using *The Happiest Toddler* tricks (the *Fast-Food Rule, Toddler-ese, playing the boob, patience-stretching*) all day long boosts daytime cooperation and cuts nighttime struggles.

■ "Side-door" lessons (including *gossiping,* doll play, and fairy tales) help you and bedtime battles.

■ Read your homemade *Beddy-Bye* book will teach your tot that sleepy-time is fun and cozy.

■ If your tot wants to play until midnight, start giving signals an hour before bedtime that sleepy-time is coming—dim lights, soft white noise, no roughhousing, no TV.

■ *Bedtime sweet talk* is a great way to end the day: giving gratitude for the joys of the day and building hope and optimism for what tomorrow will bring.

■ Family meetings and fair (*win-win*) compromises and incentives like star charts can tip the scales in your favor. This "give a little, get a little" approach will teach your child the value of compromise—*and* make bedtime easier.

■ *Twinkle interruptus* is my favorite *no-cry* sleep-training technique. It's based on *patience-stretching,* white noise, loveys . . . and love.

■ For tenacious tykes who refuse to stay tucked in, try putting their demands "on hold," another *no-tears* twist on *patience-stretching.*

## CHAPTER TWELVE

Helping Your Tyke Sleep All Night: One to Five Years

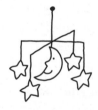

KEY POINTS:

★ **From hunger to growing pains to pinworms, several irritants can knock your tot out of dreamland.**

★ **Witches! Monsters! To a young child, these scary things are very real—and lead to sleepless nights. Luckily, you can help fears evaporate by using role-playing, fairy tales, and a little touch of magic.**

★ **Weaning from night nursing and bed-sharing can earn you extra hours of sleep. One trick that can work is to put your tot's feeding requests "on hold."**

* Picking the wrong bedtime—too late or too early— can also disturb your child's sleep.

* Learn how to help your early riser to stay asleep a little longer . . . or get your sleepyhead to wake up a little earlier.

* Sleep talking, sleepwalking, and even night terrors can all appear at this age. They're perfectly normal, but some practical steps can help chase them away.

> *Raising kids is part joy and part guerrilla warfare.*
>
> —ED ASNER

"Wake Up, Mommy!"—Oh No, Not Again!

Gigi was always a great sleeper. By five months of age, she conked out for twelve straight hours, from 7 P.M. to 7 A.M. "She was the envy of all our friends," Gigi's mom, Anita, reminisced wistfully.

But at eighteen months, that wonderful pattern came to a screeching halt. Gigi started to wake two, three, four times a night. And scream!

Anita and her husband, Paul, now drag themselves out of bed and rock Gigi back to sleep, only to be roused again from deepest slumber a few hours later. When they rock her until she falls asleep, she jolts awake the minute they lay her down on the bed. Some nights they start at 7 and don't get her down until nearly 11.

"She just keeps going and going," Anita confessed wearily. "But I'm a goner!"

Everyone thinks of the baby months as the time of sleep struggles, but toddlers and preschoolers have lots of problems, too. And if you don't take action, the problem is likely to get worse.

A Swiss study found night waking actually *increases* during the toddler years, with 22 percent of three-year-olds and about 50 percent of four-year-olds waking at night at least once a week. (Of course, families in this study didn't have white noise and all the other tricks you now have up your sleeve!)

Night waking might be caused by the problems you've wrestled with before, like teething, growth spurts, or your child's dependency on "hands-on" sleep cues like rocking or nursing.

But some new sleep struggles can also rear their head during these years. Your child's busy mind can become infested with worries and fears or her sleep may be jolted by night terrors or sleep apnea or even pinworms.

Are you ready to say good-bye to your tot's nighttime waking? If so, the first thing you need to do is figure out . . . what's going on?

The main reasons your tyke may be waking during the night are (1) something's disrupting her sleep, (2) she's a poor self-soother and depends on *you* to fall back to sleep, or (3) her bedtime is at the *wrong* time.

A "Pebble in the Shoe": Disturbances That Knock Kids Awake

Every sixty minutes—throughout the night—your child enters the light/drowsy part of her sleep cycle. That's when little commotions can jolt her totally awake. These disturbances can sneak into her mind from the outside world or they can originate from deep inside her body.

And like the Princess and the Pea, when your sweetie is in light sleep, it takes little—scratchy sheets, a ticking clock, the smell of new furniture, the hall light, a siren down the street—to nudge her from dozing to drama.

So get rid of as many outside distractions as you can and crank up the white noise to cover intruding sounds and other distractions you can't block. But if the night waking continues, you'll want to focus on some disturbances that might be prodding her awake from *inside* her body.

Hunger

About 80 percent of toddlers still get occasional bottle- or breast-feedings during the day, and they often want a middle-of-the-night snack as well. But *wanting* something isn't the same as *needing* it!

All toddlers have the ability to sleep a good eight- to ten-hour stretch, with a bit of milk at tuck-in and all the rest of their nourishment in the daytime. So if your angel still wakes and wants some sips at 2 A.M., here's how to help her kick the habit:

- **Boost daytime calories. Fruits and veggies are healthy, but low in calories. So supplement her diet with some high-cal avocado, nut butter, or olive or flaxseed meal or oil, *plus* three cups of milk or other dairy foods a day.**

- **Stop mealtime distractions, like TV, so your little one stays focused on eating.**

- **Give milk or a little food at bedtime (an egg or avocado mixed with olive oil) or wake your child up for a *dream feed* of milk at 11 P.M. (see page 168).**

- **Cut nighttime calories. Limit feedings between midnight and 6 A.M. to nursing on just one side, or if you bottle-feed, dilute the milk (give six ounces of milk with two ounces of water, and every three days reduce the milk by two ounces and add two more ounces of water). Your child will be hungrier in the morning and eat more during the day—and less at night.**

- **Use a rough white noise—all night—to distract her from mild hunger.**

- **Consider leaving a bottle in the bed. Remember, though, that leaving a bottle of cold milk or juice in the bed is a risk because some kids "comfort suck"—keep the bottle in the mouth for an hour—which can cause serious decay of the upper teeth. Instead, just leave a bottle filled with some naturally sweet, sugar-free peppermint or chamomile herbal tea.**

Teething

When those toddler canines and molars come in, it can be miserable. Like a mild headache, teething is typically easy to ignore in the daytime but can really throb at night.

If you suspect teething is causing night waking, first use a rougher white noise (as loud as a shower) to distract your little trouper from her swollen gums. (If you haven't used white noise recently, start it slowly as described on page 72.) Also ask your health-care provider about using acetaminophen or ibuprofen half an hour before bedtime.

An old-time teething remedy is to dip the corner of a thin washcloth in apple juice and freeze it. Then let your child chew on the frozen cloth.

Hard Poop and Digestive Woes

Constipation can make kids grumpy and miserable. And when your child's intestines strain to expel a hard stool at night, it can wake him up.

If you think your sweetie has a poop problem, make sure he gets plenty of exercise and water and ask your doctor for dietary recommendations, like reducing constipating foods (bread, dairy, rice, pasta, and fried food) and boosting high-fiber foods (vegetables, beans, dried fruit, and juices like prune, carrot, or aloe vera).

Dry Throat and Stuffy Nose

Little kids get lots of colds. So you can be sure your tot will occasionally have sleep troubles because of a scratchy throat or stuffy nose. (Both problems are especially common in high altitudes and desert climates, or when you're running the heater on cold winter nights.)

When that happens to your child, place a folded towel under the mattress to raise the head of the bed (unfortunately this doesn't work well if your tot flips all around during sleep) and run a cool mist humidifier all night. Use only distilled water, and clean the humidifier every day to prevent bacterial growth.

Warning: Avoid using a hot water vaporizer. It can burn your child if he touches the steam.

Try a little squirt of pure saline spray—available over the counter in any pharmacy—in each nostril. Also, soothe a cough with a syrup made with a few tablespoons of warm water mixed with a little honey and lemon juice (lemon juice has natural decongestants). One study of over 100 children found that honey was more effective than dextromethorphan (the key ingredient in medicines like Robitussin) for night cough.

If a cough persists or is spasmodic or wheezy, ask your doctor about asthma. And if your child snores or sleeps with his neck extended, ask your doctor if sleep-disordered breathing (SDB) might be the culprit. See chapter 15 for more info on both conditions.

Grandma Used Vicks VapoRub . . . Will You? Maybe Not

This century-old, over-the-counter salve has been slathered on sniffling kids for generations to open their breathing passages and warm their chests. It was a really big seller during the influenza epidemic of 1918 and for decades was touted by its manufacturer as "the only thing more powerful than a mother's touch."

But a study in 2009 found that Vicks VapoRub actually increased mucus production and inflammation and could worsen breathing problems in children under two. The manufacturer no longer recommends it for children under two years old.

I've also had young patients who accidentally rubbed some of this salve into their eyes and had terrible burning pain. Ouch!

Pinworms: Itchy Little White Threads

This is a problem that's most common at the toddler and pre-school stage. These half-inch, threadlike worms are harmless, but they can be the cause of sleep problems that come out of nowhere.

Usually, a child suddenly awakens twenty to forty minutes after falling asleep, crying or even screaming, and complaining of rectal itching or pain.

Here's how to check for these creepy crawlers. It sounds disgusting . . . but when your sweetie wakes up, bring in a flashlight and look at his anus. You may see little white threadlike worms. If so, you can put some soothing ointment on his bottom (and then wash your hands). And call the doctor in the morning.

Even if you never see the worms, a nighttime itchy anus may be a sign of this problem. Ask your doctor if medication would be warranted for your child *and all family members,* except babies. Pinworms are very easy to spread, and you don't want them to ping-pong back and forth between family members for months. (Pinworms also spread quickly in day-care settings. Be sure to tell your school about the worms, so other parents can be informed.)

The next morning—after taking the medicine—immediately give your tot a good washing. Scrub his bottom *and* his finger-nails, too, because scratching the anus will deposit microscopic eggs under the nails where they can later be spread to toys and other people.

Then, wash your child's sheets, blanket, and pillowcase in hot soapy water to rid them of any eggs.

Growing Pains and Other Leg Complaints

Miguel woke up every night just an hour after going to sleep, crying that his leg hurt. Sometimes he said his thigh ached, and other times he complained about his shin. And sometimes it was the right leg, while other times it was the left. He'd go back to sleep only after his mom gave him a little ibuprofen and massaged his leg for ten minutes.

Growing pains aren't just a myth. They affect up to 25 percent of children, generally between the ages of three and twelve. These deep pains are felt in the thigh or calf and can occur many nights a week—for months—before they just disappear.

Even though they're common, we have no clear idea what causes these aches. Are they really from *growing*—or from the jumping, climbing, and running that normal kids do all day? We just don't know. (For some children, the pains do seem to happen after very active days.)

If your child is complaining of pain at night, call your doctor. The doctor should ask you some key questions to figure out if these are routine growing pains—or something more serious:

- **Does pain or limping occur during the day?**
- **Is the pain in a joint?**
- **Is it always in the same spot on the same leg?**
- **Is the leg painful to touch?**
- **Is there any redness or swelling?**

If the answer to any of these questions is yes, then the problem is not a simple case of growing pains. The treatment of growing pains is simple and includes massage, stretching, a heating pad, and ibuprofen or another pain reliever.

Note: Another type of nighttime leg pain your tot might experience is muscle cramping. Some kids get painful spasms in their feet or legs during sleep (some adults get these, too). The cramp makes the toes curl painfully and you may be able to feel the knotted muscle in your child's calf.

The best treatment for muscle cramping is to stretch the muscle by having your child walk or firmly pushing the toes up, to stretch the calf and Achilles tendon. If this occurs more than once, a preventive remedy is to give a magnesium supplement mixed into warm milk at dinner or bedtime (this also can cause some loose stools). Ask your health-care professional for the correct dose of magnesium for your child's weight.

Fears: A Terrible Disturbance—of the Mind

Billy was four years old and always a little anxious. He'd watch other kids for weeks before he screwed up the courage to try a new swing or slide. And he hated loud noises like fireworks.

It took Billy ninety minutes to fall asleep each night. He never had a teddy as a little toddler, but insisted on holding his mom's hand until he fell asleep.

Billy's mom tried the "crying it out" technique once when he was two and a half, under pressure from her family. He cried for two hours and took two giant steps backward, becoming much more anxious for months about separating from his mom!

Over time, Billy gradually got better and his bedtime routine eventually dropped to thirty minutes.

But one night while he was sleeping, his dad burned some toast and set off the smoke alarm. Billy woke sobbing in panic. After that, his routine went back to ninety minutes, and he needed to hold his mom's hand again for almost five weeks.

Few grown-ups can remember being one year old, in a dark room, alone and terrified of being separated from Mom and Dad. But from a little kid's point of view, it must be very scary.

As your toddler toddles away and begins exploring the world, it must be bewildering—and frightening—to suddenly turn around and find yourself all alone. That's especially true for sensitive and cautious tots, like Billy. No wonder "Where's Mommy?" can suddenly escalate into a tidal wave of terror: "WHERE'S MOMMY?!!"

Separation anxiety is very, very common. It peaks at fifteen to thirty months. It's especially common after trips, illnesses, or big changes like a move, new school, or new baby.

But separation isn't the only fear that grips little kids. By the time your angel reaches two or three, he'll encounter many more things to worry about, from thunder to mean dogs to monsters, dinosaurs, and bugs.

And it doesn't stop there. At three to four years new worries just keep coming! Three-year-olds increasingly realize that they're smaller, weaker, and slower than *everybody* (except a "dumb little baby"). No wonder they suddenly start to fret about robbers, witches, and bad people.

New worries may also be triggered when a child feels anger or pressure from his parents (for instance, because of difficulties with toilet training).

Older toddlers also experience fears because of something called *projection*. They know they shouldn't bite or hit, but the desire to do so may still *well up* inside. So to push away their temptation to "do something bad," they *project* the urge from themselves onto an assortment of imaginary meanies. ("The monster took my toys, and he tried to bite me!")

Cautious kids have more fears—and these fears are usually worse and last longer. (On the other hand, you may wish your bouncy, confident tot were a little more afraid . . . so he wouldn't try jumping off the playground slide just for fun!)

Whatever the reason, young children have a new sense of vulnerability that can trigger worries that were never there before. The key to helping any child get over these fears is to go at his pace, boosting his confidence in sure, steady baby steps. Here are some ways to make the process a success.

Start by Acknowledging the Fear . . . Without Judgment

When your child shares her fears with you, don't immediately discount them. ("Honey, it's just a bad dream—see, there are no bad men in the closet.") And certainly don't roll your eyes or laugh, or call her a scaredy-cat!

Why? Because pushing children to confront their fears or belittling their worries can turn fears into panic.

That shouldn't surprise you. Fears are often irrational. They might not actually exist in the world, but they're very real in our imagination. And the harder we're pushed, the more scared, stressed, and fearful we become.

That's also why using logic to quell your tot's fear is usually a big flop ("Honey, there are no monsters in real life!"). Logic works no better with frightened kids than with frightened adults. (Imagine tying to wave away someone's fear of flying by explaining that more people die in car accidents than in plane crashes.)

So the best way to help your fearful child is to repeat back what she's telling you. Use your best *Fast-Food Rule* and *Toddler-ese* (see pages 211 and 212) to offer some sincere acknowledgment that shows that you're on her side and you "get it" ("That ghost looked really scary, huh? I didn't like her scary voice . . . what part was scary to you?").

Later, after she calms, she'll be better able to hear your reassurance: "Mommy and Daddy are here, and we'll keep you safe. Let's keep your dolly here with you, too. And would you like me to keep the light on in the hall?"

Boost Confidence During the Day

Scary things are less frightening when the sun is shining, so daytime is a perfect time to help your sweetie practice facing his fears and being brave. And there are *tons* of fun ways to do this:

GOSSIP

Let your child overhear you *gossiping* to his teddy that you are happy he shared his worries with you. And *gossip* about his little acts of bravery—for example, petting a neighbor's puppy or climbing up the slide.

ROLE-PLAY

Take turns with your child pretending to be afraid. For example, pretend that *you* are a little child, and your tot is a dog. Let him be big and scary at first, and start out frightened yourself, but see if you can end up becoming friends and helping each other. (For example, pretend the dog is scared of shadows. You can say, "Oh, you silly doggy! Bobby's not scared of shadows . . . see? Bobby can run right through them!")

Let your sweetie decide if he wants to be the kid (who tells the mean doggie that it's not nice to be scary to kids and he should learn to shake hands, not bite) or if he wants to be the dog (who can bark and yell, but who gets reminded that he'll get a time-out and no one will want to play with him if he's mean).

USE DOLL PLAY

If your child is scared of being alone, role-play this as well. Let one dolly be the mommy and the other the worried toddler. Say, "I miss Mommy. Mommy! Mommy! Mommy!! I want Mommy!!!" Then let the dolly see Mommy and say, "Oh! There you are! I knew you always come back!"

If your child is afraid of thunder, take turns making a thunder-like sound by rattling a sheet of tinfoil. Make your own storms, and have the dolls take turns being the scary storm and being the brave child.

TELL FAIRY TALES

Make up fairy tales like this one: "Once upon a time, there was a little girl froggy who was worried when her mommy hopped away from their lily pad. But she had a talking teddy bear who sang songs with her and kept her happy and safe until her mommy came back with kisses and big juicy flies to eat!"

READ BOOKS

Read your child reassuring books about things that scare her. Rachel, for instance, got a book all about ants to read to Rooney. "See, honey? See how tiny a bug is, and look how big you are! And bugs eat leaves. They think kids taste yucky! Phooey!" After they read the story, Rachel would draw a picture of a bug and let Rooney crumple it up and throw it away, saying, "Bad bug! Go away! Don't scare Rooney!"

FIND CREATIVE SOLUTIONS

Just as we might feel more secure with a can of pepper spray when we're in a dark alley, kids feel more secure with some tangible defenses. So ask your child, "What would you like better to keep you safe—your teddy, or a little flashlight?" One child was afraid of monsters under the bed, so she and dad decided to put boxes under the bed so no monsters could fit there!

Also, put a picture of your family by the bed. Or tape up a crayon drawing you made together of a kid sticking out her tongue to tell the bad guys to go away.

USE "TWINKLE INTERRUPTUS"

Last but not least, use *twinkle interruptus* (see page 255). Remember four-year-old Billy, whom I talked about at the beginning of this section—the little guy who had to fall asleep holding his mom's hand? This worked wonders with him.

At first, Billy's mom announced she had to leave the room for just two or three seconds, saying, "Wait! Wait! I'll be right back! I have to tell Daddy something important." Later that night, she did it again for ten seconds . . . and still later for fifteen seconds. Each time she left, she had her worried little boy hold her cashmere scarf.

Every night, she stretched out her absences a little longer. By the fourth night, she was planning on leaving the room for twenty, fifty, and then ninety seconds . . . but Billy fell asleep during the first twenty seconds, clutching the scarf and listening to white noise.

Twinkle interruptus and all the other approaches I've mentioned will help your little one ward off worries in the middle of the night. And one more great trick for calming fear is using the power of . . . magic!

Try a Magic Act!

To help three-year-old Marjorie deal with her fear of monsters coming into the house, her mom ended the bedtime routine with a few squirts of "secret super-spray" to give her happy dreams all night. She also put garlic on Marjorie's window because monsters run away when they smell garlic. She'd say, "Marjorie, do you know what I just remembered? Dinosaurs hate the smell of garlic. They say, 'Yucky . . . poop!' Oh! And I have a really delicious piece of stinky garlic in the refrigerator. Let's rub a tiny bit on a piece of paper and put it by the window. That will keep them away for sure!"

Magic is one of my favorite ways to boost a child's courage. That's because *secret* and *magic* are two little words that make toddlers and preschoolers feel powerful.

After all, magic is *real* to little kids. They still believe in Santa and the Easter Bunny! In their minds, a magic spell or a rock with superpowers is real protection.

So reassure your fearful friend by giving her a magic trinket that you have invested with your special mommy or daddy power (like a bracelet, a piece of a scarf, or a glove or hat). Tell her to keep it in her pocket and to touch or look at it whenever she wants to feel that you're near.

Or end your bedtime routine with a magic spell ("Abracadabra, alakazaam, monsters go home. . . . Don't come where I am!"), a magic song ("Mommy loves you, Daddy loves you, Lily is safe, safe, safe!"), or a magic spray (water with a tiny bit of orange oil in a small spray bottle with a smiley-face sticker).

And finally, what could be better than a magic suit? Tell your tot, "Let's put on your invisible supermagic suit every night, and

> that way the monsters won't be able to see you. Let's practice now." Then touch him all the way from the top of his head to his toes . . . slowly applying the invisible suit . . . making a big deal about getting every spot. Ask, "Did I get your ears? Did I miss any spots?"

Check for Legitimate Worries

Even the most cheerful little kids have fears. But if your child's fears suddenly pop up out of nowhere, try to figure out if there are problems you need to address. Is there a bully at preschool . . . or is the new babysitter mean? Was your tyke traumatized by a big storm or an earthquake? Did she watch a scary movie, or hear you and your partner arguing? Did she overhear you talking about a burglary in the neighborhood? Or is a relative abusing her?

You can also ask your child what she's afraid of, but don't push too hard for an answer. Kids often have a hard time expressing their fears.

If your tot is in preschool, ask the teachers how things are going there. And if your child has a major case of separation anxiety, try spending some time with her in the classroom.

Also, back off on pressures that may be stressing your child, like toilet training. And make sure your bedtime isn't too late, because some kids get more fearful when they're overtired.

If your child's fears are getting worse or affecting her daytime behavior, speak with your health-care provider about doing a more thorough evaluation with a child therapist. Red flags include extreme separation anxiety, excessive thumb sucking, or a return to wetting or soiling after mastering using the potty. If your child is getting into more fights, or being more defiant and disruptive, that's also a concern.

Weaning Sleep Cues That Can Slow Self-Soothing

We're all creatures of habit, and that's true for little kids as well.

Rocking and nursing are no problem if you stay with your sweetie until she falls asleep . . . as long as she sleeps through the night. In fact, about 40 percent of parents of toddlers and preschoolers cuddle like this each night.

But a child who is always rocked or nursed to sleep may get upset when she wakes up—all alone—in the middle of the night. "Hey, why did you leave? I *need* your help again!"

So, if your little bug wakes during the night and can't get back to sleep without your help, it may be time for her to become a little more independent.

In particular, research shows that between eighteen and thirty months, the following habits are linked to poor sleep:

- **Feeding your child when she wakes up during the night**
- **Taking your child out of bed to rock her**
- **Bringing your child into your bed**

One-year-olds who still nurse and bed-share often have frequent awakenings. And at two years of age, kids who nurse and bed-share wake about every 4.8 hours. Those who nurse but don't bed-share wake after about 6.9 hours, and bottle-fed babies who don't bed-share wake after about 9.5 hours.

Of course, the key to stopping bad habits is to avoid them before they start. That means waking an infant—a tiny bit—every time she's placed down to sleep (the *wake-and-sleep* technique). Parents who do that can happily rock and nurse their small friends into profound relaxation and still help them develop their self-soothing skill.

But, if you're reading this section, it probably means you missed the boat during the early months and you're now trying to figure out how to get back on track and wean your older child off needing your help to soothe herself back to sleep each time she wakes.

Fortunately, there are still many things you can do to lovingly boost your child's independence and help both of you sleep longer and better. Here's how.

Weaning Night Feeding (Bottle or Breast): Put Your Tot's Request "On Hold"

Feeding your toddler one to three times a night is perfectly fine and normal. It's how our ancestors did it for thousands of years.

However, those ancestors didn't need to rush to the office for a 9 A.M. meeting—and they had tons of friends and family to help with child care and daily chores! In today's world, losing sleep every night can be grueling or (when you're on the road) even dangerous.

Fortunately, one-year-olds can easily be weaned from night feeds—even night nursing. (Amazingly, your breasts can automatically boost milk production during the day and slow it down at night.)

You'll know your tot is ready to stop night feeds when he drinks just an ounce or two from the bottle or sucks at the breast for a minute or two and then dozes off again. This tells you he doesn't really *need* to eat at night, he's using you more as a pacifier.

To bring these inconvenient meals to a happy end for the baby and you, you'll need to do a little work in the daytime and at night.

In the Daytime . . .

Practice all the methods you learned earlier to increase your child's feelings of confidence, ability to be patient, and desire to cooperate: *patience-stretching, magic breathing,* a star chart, role-play, your *Beddy-Bye* book, and so on (see pages 213–18 and 238).

At Night . . .

Set a regular bedtime with a nice routine of sleep cues: white noise all night, a lovey, a night-light, and a little lavender oil to scent the bed. Make sure you leave the room while your child is still awake.

When your little bug wakes in the middle of the night, sending Daddy in for the 2 A.M. cuddle may help her be comforted without needing to nurse.

However, if she continues to wake for feedings, try putting her demand "on hold" (see page 257). Here's how.

First, spend a week practicing *patience-stretching* during the day and using white noise all night.

Then, when she wakes at 2 A.M., comfort her right away, but delay feeding her for a minute or two (if you can). And as you bring the bottle—or begin opening your nightgown—to feed her, suddenly raise a finger and exclaim, "Wait! Wait! One second, sweetheart!" and quickly go across the room, pretending to look for something. Return in five seconds, and then do the feeding.

Over the course of the next week, gradually stretch the time you pretend to be searching to several minutes, until your tot starts falling asleep while she's waiting.

If your little one gets upset, come right back and almost feed her again, but at the last second say, "Oh, silly Mommy, I forgot to tell Daddy something! Be right back, honey!" and leave again for a short time.

Is this tricky? Yes, but it works! Remember, your child doesn't really *need* nighttime feedings anymore. Her waking is just the residue of an old habit.

Weaning Your Tot from Bed-Sharing

In an article by Laura Stampler on the Huffington Post website, Cindy confessed that she and her husband bed-share. "I'm sleeping with another man," she said. "Two men actually. Two men and a dog. But the dog sleeps on the floor." Noting that she's a working mom, Cindy said, "If I didn't sleep with [my son], I might just see him for one or two hours in a day."

In the same article, Morgan was less enthusiastic about sharing the covers with his kids. He described how he and his wife have been trying to wean their children from their bed—but each time, their efforts are met with screaming fits and ultimately they cave.

"I hate it, and so does my wife," Morgan said. "It's awkward that we sleep with our kids rather than each other. They kick, and when my two-year-old is tired he grabs my ear, and he's made it bleed."

We're used to thinking of bed-sharing as something parents do with nursing babies, but it starts happening all over again once kids pass two years of age. It may start during a vacation, an illness, or a stressful time (new school, new house, divorce, etc.). And surprisingly, bed-sharing (at least once a week) peaks at four years of age.

Bed-sharing with your toddler or preschooler can be a really wonderful experience as long as you're not doing it for the wrong reasons (such as avoiding intimacy with your partner)—and as long as you and your partner *both* like sharing the bed with your little one.

In a recent study, researchers looked at 944 families (mostly Hispanics and African Americans) and found that bed-sharing toddlers had no negative cognitive or behavioral outcomes.

Bed-sharing is also much, much safer at this age than during the early months. But make sure your room is totally childproofed. Crawl everywhere and tug on everything to check. Watch out for cords, appliances, sharp corners, electric outlets, windows, sharp grills, things in the garbage can, pennies or staples on the floor, plastic bags in the closet, and so on. And never put medicine in your nightstand.

To keep everyone cozy in this arrangement, consider getting a bigger bed. Or consider putting a little bed next to yours . . . or perhaps put your mattress on the floor with a mat and sleeping bag next to it for your child.

Cozy or not, the day will eventually come when it's time to wean your child from nightly bed-sharing (although most of us continue to bed-share on occasion for many years to come). Here are some simple, gentle, and effective ways to do it.

In the Daytime . . .

Give your tyke lots of comforting routines like *special time,* a daily massage, or cookies and milk every afternoon. And build her sense of confidence by giving her options ("Should we have cereal or eggs for breakfast?") and *playing the boob* (see chapter 10).

Also, use confidence-building techniques like:

- **Playing hide-and-seek. This teaches your tot that when you go away, you always come back.**

- **Practicing *patience-stretching* and *magic breathing* to boost his ability to handle frustration and to endure short separations (see pages 213 and 214).**

- **Playing on his bed during the day to boost his familiarity and comfort with it.**

- **Gossiping. Let your child overhear you talking to his teddy or dollies about how cozy it is sleeping in his own bed.**

- **Looking at his *Beddy-Bye* book with him every day to help him build the right expectations.**

- **Acting out bedtime with his dollies (see page 238).**

At Night . . .

To many little kids, a dark bedroom can seem like a scary cave. Your tot will handle her new independence better if you can show her that it's a comfy nest instead.

First, turn off the TV . . . or better yet, keep it out of her room altogether. Children with a TV in their bedroom are twice as likely to have nighttime fears!

Next, ease the transition to night by dimming the lights and playing soft white noise (like rain on the roof) an hour before bedtime so the switch from bright light to darkness is not so abrupt: give massages, sing lullabies, do *bedtime sweet talk*, and use a lovey.

For the first three or four nights, sleep next to her bed all night. Once she's sleeping well in her bed, move your sleeping bag or cot two feet away from the bed. When she's okay with that, move halfway to the door for a few days . . . then next to the door . . . then just outside the door. Check in on her every ten to fifteen minutes after lights-out to reassure her that you're still thinking of her.

Once she's ready to stay in her room on her own, keep the door open. Use a gate to keep her in her room, and provide a mat, pillow, and blanket by the door in case she chooses to sleep by the door instead of in the bed.

Be flexible. You may make progress, but then have a couple of rough nights when things slide back again. That's okay. Being alone for even five minutes can be hard for a fearful child, and your most important goal is to lower your sweetie's anxiety level and help her feel safe enough to start enjoying bedtime again.

Don't make a big deal about her success! This can backfire by making your child feel more pressured because it is obviously so important to *you.* It may also make her feel like a failure if she backslides a bit. So be positive, but understated. During the day, *gossip* about her victories, but don't overdo *your* happiness about it.

Stay at home. When your angel is sleeping, she needs there to be a person whom she trusts completely (not a new babysitter). Waking up and having no one familiar to comfort her can cause her to quickly regress and send everything back to square one.

A Bedtime That's Too Late—or Too Early—May Backfire

For most tots, lights-out is around 9 P.M. (give or take thirty minutes), but pushing it later or trying to force it earlier may lead to *more* middle-of-the-night waking!

Is Bedtime Too Late?

Overtired children often get more hyper. *Rather than winding down, they get wound up!*

This leads to bedtime resistance, and the memory of these struggles can reverberate throughout the nighttime and actually wake your tot when she enters one of her light stages of sleep in the middle of the night.

Signs that your bedtime may be too late include:

■ **Your child is overactive, irritable, and accident-prone at bedtime.**

■ **She resists bedtime with all sorts of excuses, complaints, and defiant acts.**

■ **She acts tired all day (excess yawning and staring, falling asleep in the car or while snacking, etc.).**

If this seems to be the problem, the key to success is *stacking the deck* in your favor during the day!

Spend time boosting patience and cooperation during the day (perhaps even with a star chart and incentive program for going to bed—see page 215) and start a calming, *prebedtime* routine sixty minutes before your sleep routine even begins (see page 241).

And, of course, shift your tot's bedtime routine thirty minutes earlier. (Make sure it's a very enjoyable time—with loveys, white noise, *bedtime sweet talk,* etc.)

Sometimes, however, the problem isn't a bedtime that's too late . . . it's one that's too early.

Is Bedtime Too Early?

How does too early a bedtime cause night waking? For most toddlers, it's simply too much to ask for them to snooze straight through from 7 P.M. till 7 A.M. It's just more sleep than they need.

Signs that your bedtime may be too early include:

- **Your child shows no fatigue at bedtime (no yawning, blinking, staring, etc.).**

- **She repeatedly calls for you or reappears at the door for thirty to sixty minutes.**

- **She wakes in the middle of the night refreshed and ready to play.**

If this seems to be the problem, gradually shift her routine. Delay all *daytime* meals and naps by fifteen minutes, and start the bedtime routine fifteen minutes later. Then, every three days, delay all these by another fifteen minutes.

Within a week or two bedtime should be between 8 P.M. and 8:30 P.M., and your child should stop resisting your bedtime routine, fall asleep quickly, and stop waking in the middle of the night.

Early Birds and Sleepyheads

Even if your young friend falls into slumber easily and sleeps well all night, there are two last snooze hurdles that might become issues: waking too early or sleeping too late.

The average young child wakes up at 7:21 A.M., but this may range from 5:30 A.M. to 8 A.M.! About one-third of toddlers and preschoolers wake up in the morning before their parents do at least a few days a week. Here's a look at the statistics.

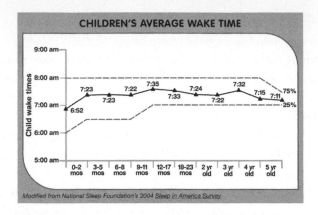

CHILDREN'S AVERAGE WAKE TIME

Modified from National Sleep Foundation's 2004 Sleep in America Survey.

It can be exhausting when your tot is getting up with the roosters. The most common reasons early birds pop awake too soon:

- **They're going to bed too early.**
- **They're napping too much.**
- **They're waking up with the morning lights and sounds.**
- **They naturally don't need very much sleep. (Yikes, God forbid!).**

If bedtime is too early, follow the instructions in the previous section. This should solve the problem quickly.

If your little guy is taking an afternoon nap that lasts more than two hours, begin shortening the nap by gently waking him fifteen minutes early. I know it never feels right to wake a sleeping toddler, but this may be the only way you can get him to wake up at a better time in the morning.

Also, waking too early may be a sign that your tot is ready to drop a nap (go from two naps to one or from one to none). So you may want to try to keep him busier during the day and see if you can nudge him into giving up the extra nap. If he gets more cranky and distraught, he probably isn't ready to make the change yet.

Some tots wake at the crack of dawn, as soon as light filters through the bedroom window. For these kids, using heavy shades to darken the window may delay wake-up. A rough white noise may also help them ignore the light.

And finally, some kids just inherit a need for less sleep. Like adults who are fine with six hours of sleep each night, these little guys feel just peachy with ten hours a day instead of twelve to fourteen.

If your child continues to wake at 5 A.M. despite all your efforts, these tricks may buy you a little extra sleep:

- Encourage him to play by himself by giving him some favorite toys, warm milk, and lullaby music (or even a special DVD) that he only gets to play with during these morning hours.

- Make a fun spot in the room (a tent or cardboard box cave with pillows and toys inside) that can be a special place for him to lounge in the early morning with a warm bottle of milk.

- Practice *patience-stretching* and *magic breathing*, and use sticker charts or poker chips to encourage him to learn to be patient and stay in his room. (See pages 213–17.)

- Change your white noise. Try a rougher sound, like a hair dryer sound or a CD of rain on the roof.

- Bring your tot into your bed for a cozy final hour of sleep.

But maybe you have the opposite problem. Does your tot like rock-star hours—bedding down at 12 A.M. and sleeping till 10 A.M.? About 10 percent of toddler parents and 20 percent of preschooler parents complain that their kids have real difficulty waking in the morning.

The most common reasons children wake up too late are:

- They're going to bed too late.

- They have very disturbed sleep.

- They're not napping enough.

- They naturally need a lot of sleep.

If bedtime is too late—after 9:30 P.M.—the strategies I outlined in the previous section will help you solve the problem. (See page 284.)

Also, make sure your child is getting lots of sunlight and fresh air during the day and no caffeine. And give her brain the signal that sleepy-time is getting closer by dimming the lights, playing white noise, and reducing exciting play and TV an hour before her bedtime routine starts.

You might also ask your doctor about using a little melatonin (see page 135) after dinner for a week or two, to shift her circadian sleep cycle a little earlier.

If your little sleepyhead is exhausted even though she's going to bed at a good time, maybe her sleep is being broken by many short awakenings all through the night. This could be due to outside disturbances, but it could also be due to some of the medical problems, like asthma or sleep apnea, that I discuss in chapter 15.

And what if it's hard to get your tot down for a nap because your day is so hectic, or because she's almost outgrown napping? Then she just might *need* that extra sixty minutes of sleep in the morning. If that's the case, and you don't work outside the home, let her enjoy it . . . and take advantage of that extra hour to get some exercise, catch up on chores, or relax a little yourself!

Bizarre Behaviors: From Nightmares to Night Terrors

The toddler and preschool years can also see the start of strange sleep disturbances, like sleep talking and night terrors. I mentioned these oddities of sleep—also called *parasomnias*—back in chapter 1 (see page 20). Most of these occur during NREM sleep when part of your child's brain stays anchored in very deep sleep, while other parts are bubbling back up to light sleep.

Now let's take a closer look at these alarming, but totally normal and benign, events in the deep of night.

Sleepwalking—Very Odd to Watch

Sleep talking and sleepwalking can throw you for a loop if you're not expecting them.

In sleep talking, kids calmly sit up in bed—*eyes open, but glassy*—and start speaking in short, incoherent phrases. Your child may stop if you call her, turn to you, and mumble some gibberish (some older kids actually say clear phrases like "No, no, go away!"), but she won't look you in the eyes. In fact, she'll seem to be looking right through you!

While many parents take sleep talking in stride, sleep*walking* can be a bit worrisome. There your child is, moving around the room—eyes open—as if looking for something, searching in a closet or toy box . . . or walking into the hall . . . even trying to get out of the house! . . . yet totally in "la-la" land.

Sleepwalking occurs in up to 20 percent of children and can begin as early as the toddler years (although it's most common between eight and twelve years of age). It may go on for months or years.

Episodes typically last five to fifteen minutes and occur during the first couple of hours of sleep. Sleepwalkers are very hard to wake up and usually just return to bed for a deep, peaceful sleep or end up waking up confused with no recollection of the episode.

Thankfully, it's rare for sleepwalkers to fall and get hurt. Nevertheless, parents have occasionally found their kids on the front lawn trying to get out the gate . . . eyes open, but totally asleep! So you'll want to latch the doors and windows and use a gate or a slippery doorknob cover so your sweetie can't easily get out—or at least put a bell on her door.

If you catch your tot sleepwalking, calmly steer her back to bed, speaking very little and in a soft voice. Singing often seems to soothe these little zombies more than talking—so when the parasomnia occurs, make your white noise a little louder and sing a familiar lullaby over and over to get her back into bed.

These episodes are hard to stop, but here are a few tricks that might help you reduce them a little. First, avoid giving your child chocolate or other stimulants, including antihistamines, decongestants, and caffeine-containing drinks. Second, see if you can extend her sleep (longer naps, earlier bedtimes). Third, if sleep talking or sleepwalking is happening every night, wake your child one hour after she falls asleep. (This may stop the parasomnia by resetting the sleep cycle.)

Tooth Grinding— Another Bizarre Sleep Event

Ugh! Listening to your two-year-old scraping her upper and lower teeth together can be even more disturbing than hearing fingernails scratch across a chalkboard.

Contrary to the old wives' tale, tooth grinding isn't a sign of intestinal worms. It's just another one of the weird problems that can occur during deep NREM sleep.

Tooth grinding, or bruxism, can start as early as the first birthday and cause sleep disruption, tooth wear (even fractures), and jaw pain. It can be provoked by caffeine-containing food and drinks like chocolate, iced tea, and cola. And it's especially common among kids with obvious neurological disorders, like cerebral palsy.

Most kids outgrow tooth grinding by the teen years. In the meantime, stress-reducing bedtime routines can reduce the problem. Sometimes doctors also prescribe mouth guards.

Confusional Arousals and Night Terrors

Confusional arousals are just what they sound like. Your child may mumble or sob and thrash about seeming upset or even agitated. He may even cry out and push you away, saying, "No, no! I don't like it!" These episodes usually last for just a minute or two and then end with your child returning to deep sleep.

Sleep terrors or *night terrors* are an extreme version of confusional arousals.

These are scary to witness. Your child may cry out—or scream—arching his back, his face filled with panic. He may be sweating, with a heaving chest and racing heart, staring into the darkness, yet totally unaware of your presence!

Parents get confused because these kids look almost awake but they're *totally* unreachable. That's because in reality, they're deep in sleep.

We call these *terrors,* but we don't even know if children are experiencing the type of fear we call terror. What we *do* know is that nothing parents do during an episode seems to help. These disruptions last five to fifteen minutes (or occasionally longer). In the end, kids just fall back to sleep or awaken, dazed, with no recollection of the event. Parents, on the other hand, may be totally traumatized for hours!

Unlike sleep talking and sleepwalking, confusional arousals are more common among children under five years of age. Sleep terrors occur in about one in twenty children—rarely as young as four years of age, but usually school age or older. Parasomnias tend to run in families . . . so if you scared the daylights out of your parents with sleep terrors, they may be getting their revenge now!

It's reassuring to know that these odd events pose no danger. But they're no fun for you, so here are some tricks that may help keep them at bay.

First, steer clear of the stimulants I talked about earlier. Also, try to reduce your child's life stresses (including violent TV, video, and cartoons).

Keep to your regular nap and nighttime schedule (going to bed too late can be a provocation). Use a strong white noise all night. During your *bedtime sweet talk*, mention how your sweetie's brain can be so relaxed he will probably have very happy dreams and sleep beautifully all the way till morning. You might even add a drop or two of lavender oil on the mattress.

During an episode, turn up the white noise (to the level of a loud shower), sing a familiar lullaby, or just repeat simple words like "You're safe, you're safe, Daddy's here . . . Daddy's here." Eventually, your child will lie back down asleep again.

If your child has had one of these sleep disturbances, caution your mom or the babysitter about this before leaving your child in their care. But don't talk to others about it in front of your child, because it may confuse or embarrass him. And let your doctor know, especially if the disturbances happen after midnight, just so he or she can rule out other problems.

Nightmares

If sleep walking and night terrors (the NREM parasomnia) are a mix of movement and drama, nightmares (the REM parasomnia) are all drama with very little action. Remember, in REM sleep, the brain's commands to the muscles of the body can't get past a "roadblock" at the base of the brain. So even though there may be a riot of thoughts and visions going on in the dream, the body stays still, even limp (thank goodness!).

In adults, bad dreams often seem to be about old memories . . . but for toddlers, nightmares are about the threatening *here and now* (angry adults, loud trucks, mean dogs, etc.).

Unlike the sleep terrors, nightmares are definitely upsetting to children. Think about how real dreams sometimes seem to us, and imagine how real—and scary—they must seem to a toddler! They can cause a child to fear falling asleep, and even to fear being in the bedroom.

Nightmares are very common and can start as early as two to three years of age. They begin at this time for the same reasons that fears begin:

- **Kids are feeling more vulnerable.**

- **They are witnessing and experiencing more upsetting things, either in real life or on TV.**

- **They're holding back angry feelings, because we're beginning to expect them to control their aggressive impulses and not hit, bite, or yell. Those corralled thoughts and actions can break through at night into violent, scary dreams.**

In night terrors, children push their parents away or just ignore them, but in nightmares they cling to us for dear life! Some children fall back to sleep after a nightmare, but many need reassurance. So be prepared to either cozy up in your sweetie's bed or let her come into your bed for a cuddle.

If your child does remember a dream of a scary monster or animal, draw pictures of it and then let her jump up and down on them or crumple them up. Or make up a little story about Benny the Bunny having the scary dream and create an ending that's less scary. Or do some role-playing games in which you're the scared child and your child is the big monster . . . and then switch roles so she gets to be the brave child and you are the bully monster, who really is a scaredy-cat who misses her mommy!

Crib Notes:
Reviewing *The Happiest Toddler* Way

- Fears are a major sleep stealer during the toddler and preschool years. Don't just dismiss them . . . use *Happiest Toddler* techniques (like *Toddler-ese*, role-playing, fairy tales, magic, and *twinkle interruptus*) to give your tot the courage to deal with her worries.

- You can wean your tot off old habits and build her self-soothing skill by practicing the *wake-and-sleep* method.

- Wean nighttime feedings by *boosting daytime calories*, offering *dream feeds* . . . and putting your toddler's requests "on hold."

- Wean bed-sharing by using your *Beddy-Bye* book, *magic breathing* and *patience-stretching* to build your tot's confidence during the day and by making her bedroom feel cozy and welcoming at night.

## CHAPTER THIRTEEN

Q&A: The Whys About Tot and Preschooler Sleep: One to Five Years

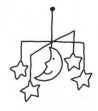

1. Why do some tots wake up so cranky?

Just as with adults, some kids seem to wake up on the *wrong side of the crib!* This is especially common with individuals who have a cautious, slow-to-warm-up temperament.

If your tyke shows signs of fatigue all day long (low energy, falling asleep in the car, dark circles under her eyes, yawning a lot, etc.), try to figure out:

- **Is her bedtime too late?**
- **Is her sleep upset by sounds, lights, or internal sleep stoppers (like teething)?**

- Is her own snoring shattering her sleep by causing frequent arousals through the night?

On the other hand, if she's grumpy on first waking but then fine the rest of the day, she's probably just hungry (some kids get übercranky when their blood sugar hits bottom in the predawn hours).

2. I can't wait to play with my eighteen-month-old when I get home at 8 P.M., but by then he's usually bleary eyed and whiny. Any ideas?

One of the great rewards of a hard day's work is to come home and play with your little child. But it sounds like the window of opportunity is almost closed by the time you arrive.

Perhaps a better idea would be to push his afternoon nap a bit later so that he's not just running on fumes when you come home. Or you might have his caretaker put him to bed when he's tired—before you get home—and have your playtime in the morning, before you go to work.

3. I rock and sing my two-year-old to sleep every night. I love it, but my pediatrician says I'm teaching him a bad habit. Should I stop?

Rocking and singing your little child into slumber is a beautiful and loving tradition. Just be aware that there are two ways your routine might lead to a little trouble:

- **You're the only one who can put him to sleep. There may be rare situations where you won't be available at your tot's bedtime (for instance, if you get sick or have to travel because of a family emergency). So encourage him to develop a good transitional relationship (loveys and familiar white noise are ideal) and to allow another caregiver to occasionally perform the bedtime routine with him.**

- **He repeatedly wakes**—*demanding that you rock him back to sleep*. **To solve this problem, make sure he's a tiny bit awake when you place him in his crib. That way, he'll learn to soothe** himself to sleep. But, if he does fall asleep before you ease him into the crib, just do the *wake-and-sleep* technique (see page 88).

4. Do you have any advice for helping my three-year-old twins sleep? They giggle and chat (or sometimes fight) for an hour after lights-out.

Having twins (or older and younger kids) share a bedroom is great for the kids. After all, who wants to sleep in a room alone? Talking to each other and being silly is one of the great memories brothers and sisters have of these quiet hours when they're the rulers of their world.

But of course, all that laughing, talking, and arguing can keep the sandman away! Here are a few tricks that can help reduce the shenanigans after the bedtime routine is over.

During the day:

- Try to get your kids outdoors for lots of sunlight, fresh air, and play (even in crummy weather).

- Practice *patience-stretching*, magic breathing, and *playing the boob* (see pages 213, 214, and 218) to boost their ability and willingness to cooperate and to help them begin learning how to resist their impulses.

- Have a family meeting to make bedtime rules. Ask your kids for their opinions and suggestions and come to a *win-win* solution. "After lights-out, should you have five minutes to quietly chat before you go to sleep, or ten minutes?" Then get their agreement that the best way to keep track is by placing a timer outside the room and setting it to ring when time is up.

- Use hand checks, a star chart system, or tokens to reward their cooperation with the new plan (see page 215).

- Sidestep bedtime battles by looking at the *Beddy-Bye* book every day, *gossiping* about their good behavior, and doing a little role-playing with their dolls to teach them the behavior you like—through the "side door" of their minds.

At *night:*

■   **Prepare their minds for sleep by dimming the lights, playing soft white noise, turning off the TV, and avoiding roughhousing for an hour before bedtime.**

■   **Offer loveys and use a strong white noise all night. Being in a stone-quiet, dark room invites kids to giggle and talk. White noise calms them and discourages conversation.**

■   **Sing or do *bedtime sweet talk* with your younger child till he falls asleep (let your older one have a flashlight and read books while you do this). Then, after the first child gets drowsy, have a quiet reading session with the older one.**

    If the younger one protests, try putting his demand "on hold" (see page 279). Acknowledge his desire and start to go back to his bed . . . then remember you have to finish reading with the older child. Start with a minute or so of this trick and keep stretching it out longer.

■   **Try not to take sides. You may see one child hitting but not know that the other was goading him into reacting.**

■   **Consider different bedtimes. You can even do it with twins. If it doesn't work, you can always return to the old routine.**

If the kids are still causing problems despite all your efforts, consider sleeping on a sleeping bag in their room for a while—or have the more challenging child move into your room to sleep in a little tent, or on a pad on the floor, for a week or two.

5. When I'm putting my two-year-old to bed, I always end up falling asleep with her for thirty minutes. Is that okay?

It's fine as long as she stays asleep till morning. However, if she wakes and needs you again at night, you should make sure you are using strong white noise all night . . . and don't forget to do the quick *wake-and-sleep* routine. Wake her up a tiny bit when you're about to leave, so she can learn to soothe herself back to sleep with the help of just white noise and a lovey.

6. When is it safe to use pillows and blankets?

SIDS is rare after six months, and the SIDS period is totally over after the first birthday. So after that, it's safe to use pillows and blankets. However, most kids sleep fine without them. So it's best to use only a blanket in the crib and add a small, flat pillow later when a child moves to a bed.

7. When my child was sick for three days, I went in to comfort him a few times each night. Now he's better, but still waking up . . . did I make a mistake?

Don't worry. When your child is sick, it's incredibly important to check on him, and it's totally normal to relax your rules. Once he recovers, you can retrain him using all the tips listed in the sleep-training section (see page 184).

8. How can I get my fifteen-month-old to let her dad put her to sleep?

The toddler years can be a mixed bag for dads. Between one and two years of age (the peak of separation worries), many kids only want Mommy to put them to sleep. But this can totally flip between two and four years! That's when lots of these little tricksters start pushing their moms away and become enraptured with playing with Daddy!

Luckily, there are ways to help your tot get comfortable being put to sleep by Daddy (or other caregivers like Grandma or the babysitter). In general, the best way to start this process is to practice during the day because you really don't want to start a big struggle right before bed. Here's what you can do:

- **Do doll play showing your tot how Daddy Bear puts Baby Bear to sleep.**

- Have Mommy *gossip* about how happy she is when your toddler lets Daddy put her to sleep.

- Have Daddy (or Grandma) play with your sweetie—a lot—and *play the boob* with her—a lot—to build rapport.

- Make sure your *Beddy-Bye* book has photos of your little munchkin playing and snuggling with Daddy.

- Use all your good sleep cues.

- Finally—and this may sound funny—make sure Daddy doesn't have a strong smell. Little kids are very sensitive to odors, so Dad should brush his teeth, wash his hands, and even carry a little piece of your clothing over his shoulder so your sweetie can catch a little of your familiar scent.

PART IV

Tips to Create Happy Naps and to Handle Special Situations

Chapter 14 tells you how to ease your tot through two big changes: the switch from two naps to one, and the end of napping altogether. In addition, I'll share my secrets for dealing with a child who catnaps, resists naps, or sleeps too long in the day and keeps you awake at night. I'll finish by answering common questions about missed naps, naptime sleep training, and more.

Chapter 15 looks at some special challenges that can

keep you and your child awake. First, I'll talk about medical problems ranging from asthma and allergies to autism and ADHD. I'll also explore the link between sleep-disordered breathing and obesity and explain why "T&A" surgery is making a big comeback. Finally, I'll offer tips for overcoming the insomnia that may keep you tossing and turning even when your little one is sound asleep.

## CHAPTER FOURTEEN

Nipping Nap Problems in the Bud

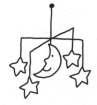

KEY POINTS:

★ Slowly your child's nap schedule will shift from twice a day, to once . . . to none. The end of naps marks your tot's passage into childhood.

★ If your infant falls asleep in your arms, always jostle her a tiny bit when you slip her into the bassinet (the *wake-and-sleep* technique).

★ The same good sleep cues (like white noise and loveys) that promote nighttime sleep work for naps, too!

* The main reasons toddlers resist naps are either because they're overtired or because they're overstimulated. Both problems are pretty easy to solve.

* Napping *too much* can lead to poor nighttime sleep, but you can take steps to shift your child's slumber back to the nighttime.

"A day without a nap is like a cupcake without frosting."
—Terri Guillemets

Naps: A Sweet (and Sacred) Time

Naps are invaluable allies when it comes to keeping your child healthy and happy. They boost his memory, restore his energy and gentle demeanor, foster his attention skills, reinvigorate his immune system, and help the stress hormones—cortisol and adrenaline—drop to low levels.

If you have a really easy child, you may be able to get away with changing his nap schedule or even skipping a nap every once in a while if you're out and about—but smart parents know to *treat naps as a sacred time.* Just as you wouldn't go out to a movie during the middle of the night, you shouldn't schedule "mommy and me" classes in the middle of your sweetie's naptime.

One by one, these blissful oases of quiet will evaporate. Yet, exactly when each of these naps will disappear is one of the least predictable aspects of your child's sleep.

3, 2, 1 . . . Blastoff: The End of Naps Marks Your Tot's Passage into Childhood

If I were to design an insignia of the early years, it would be a picture of a precious two-year-old innocently napping. Once the preschool years arrive, your child's pattern will change . . . indeed her *life* will change. She'll cross the threshold—leaving the house and entering the world—never to return to the land of naps until she has her own baby (or reaches old age).

When exactly does this momentous transition occur? The timing is different for every child, but this chart offers clues.

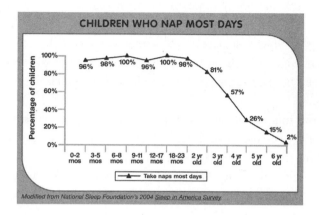

Your little one will reach this passage into childhood in a series of steps. The older she gets, the fewer naps she'll take. But as you can see in the graph below, between six and twenty-four months things can be pretty crazy! Some of these kids are still sleeping like babies while others already nap like preschoolers.

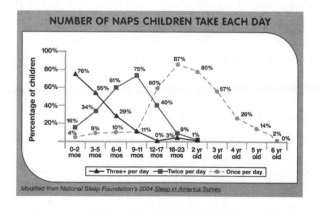

However, if we look at the averages, we can at least make some good guesses. So here's what you can expect . . . more or less.

By *three months*, your little one will have three regular and predictable naps (midmorning, midafternoon, and a short one in early evening). You'll probably organize them into a flexible schedule to help you plan your day and give your child the predictability and routine that all infants crave.

To promote your baby's self-soothing skill, make sure her eyes are open when you place her down for the nap. If she has already fallen asleep in your arms, just give her a little jostle when you deposit her in the bassinet (the *wake-and-sleep* technique . . . see page 88).

Your infant will nap much more soundly if—over the first four months—you use swaddling, rough white noise, and perhaps even rocking in a *fully reclined* swing (always ask your child's doctor for permission to do this) to help naps get established more easily.

In fact, you want to make sure your little girl is not napping too long during the day! In general, you should limit naps to two hours in duration (more or less)—especially when you are weaning your child off the afternoon nap around four or five months. Naps over three hours definitely reduce nighttime sleeping.

When you can, you, too, should try to nap during one of these peaceful periods. Many moms find it really helps *their* sleep if they block out disturbances by using white noise and an eye mask.

By *six to twelve months*, your darling will have shifted down to just two naps a day. Typically, the naps last one hour—two hours, max—but some kids are catnappers who pop back up to play after just thirty minutes. Most parents find that the two-nap schedule makes keeping to a regular schedule—the timing and duration of the naps—much easier.

By *twelve to twenty-four months*, napping will be reduced to just one a day.

As your child moves into the toddler years, you will be deeply grateful for her naps. Tots are such buzzing, bouncing bundles of energy that this hour or two of midday calm is critical for helping their parents and caregivers recover from the morning and prepare for the afternoon. You'll find that white noise and loveys continue to be invaluable aids in keeping naptime regular and successful, even when you're on a trip.

And what should you expect if your sweetie is in day care? That depends!

Some kids have trouble napping because of the distractions and come home exhausted. Others doze right off because they mimic all the other kids napping. Still others nap fine at school, but skip naps on the weekends because of all the activity going on at home.

If your tot has trouble napping at school, use her white noise and cuddly lovey there, too.

Is Your Tot Ready to Go from Two Naps to One?

Some parents proudly look at the change from two naps to one as a major accomplishment, something akin to a college graduation! But what's the rush? Daytime naps are lovely, and as I've said, adequate daytime sleep promotes good nighttime sleep—*sleep begets sleep*. Although it is also true that *too much* daytime sleep may delay bedtime or cause middle-of-the-night waking.

Most tots give up the second nap between twelve and twenty-four months. But be aware, this transition period is often rocky. Some toddlers give up the morning nap, some the afternoon nap . . . and others alternate (one day they nap in the morning, the next day in the afternoon)!

Consider yourself very lucky if your little guy is happy and playful in the late morning as he starts to skip his postbreakfast snooze. More often, tots start skipping the morning nap *but still need it*. And this internal ambivalence makes them overtired and extra grumpy . . . and weepy. (In other words, even more like a little *caveman* than usual!)

Your little man may spend a few weeks bouncing back and forth between one and two naps. (It's almost like he needs one and a half naps per day!) Many parents find that the best strategy for this "in between" period is to at least have a midmorning rest time (with white noise, a lovey, and perhaps a little reading or massage). If your child seems antsy, let him watch twenty minutes of a *calm*ing Sesame Street or nature DVD (no cartoons, please).

If your little guy switches to one nap, but then starts waking too early in the morning and seems overtired all day (irritable, staring, rubbing his eyes, falling asleep while snacking, being more clumsy, etc.), go back to two naps for a month or two.

When he finally settles into a one-nap schedule, the noon nap will last a little longer, and lunch, dinner, and bedtime will arrive a little earlier.

Is Your Tot Ready to Go from One Nap to None?

Like big, clumsy birds that plop back to the earth a few times as they run, trying to get airborne, some toddlers take many weeks—bouncing along—before they're definitely able to take flight and say au revoir to their last nap. They struggle to stay awake during play and fall fast asleep the instant they're put in the car. And they become wild during afternoon play—melting into tearful streams of "no, no, no!"—yet keel over in the high chair before they get even halfway through dinner.

About 20 percent of two-year-olds have stopped all naps—although you can be sure those parents wish they still had that little break during the day! By the third birthday, 43 percent of kids no longer nap. And that increases to 74 percent of four-year-olds and 85 percent of five-year-olds.

An early sign that the nap is waning is when your child sleeps at preschool but skips it on the weekend.

Most kids take this final step over several weeks—napping some days and not others. Ultimately, your child will completely switch to an afternoon *quiet time.*

When your tyke gives up her last nap, expect her to start running out of gas earlier in the evening. *So be prepared to slide dinner and bedtime an hour earlier.*

Surprisingly, your four-year-old will go to bed earlier than she did at eighteen months! But that's what she must do to continue getting ten to twelve hours of sleep a day after napping is finished. (And don't be surprised if, during this transition, your lovebug also pops awake in the morning a little earlier than usual.)

Common Nap Problems and How to Solve Them

Some kids sleep too little during the day, some too much, and some just sleep at the wrong time. But, by far and away, the most distressing of these is *napping too little.*

Your little cave-kid may struggle so much with naps that his room starts to feel to you like an Ultimate Fighting ring. The main reasons your tot may try to wriggle out of his nap are:

- **He's overtired.**
- **He's distracted and overstimulated (by noise, light, the TV, roughhousing, caffeine, or medications).**

Here's a quick look at each problem and how to solve it.

Overtired—"I'm Worn Out!"

The ultimate sign of whether your little ballerina is napping enough is how tired she gets during the day. Is she: Falling asleep in the car? Slumping over well before naptime arrives? Cranky and bleary eyed at dinnertime?

If so, try putting her down twenty minutes earlier for the nap. Many kids just do better if they're put down after two or three hours of play—*even if they don't seem sleepy.*

Think of this as like eating lunch before you're really hungry. Often when you sit down to eat, you realize, "Hmm . . . I didn't know it, but I guess I *am* hungry!" Similarly, anticipating your tot's need for sleep can keep her a happy napper.

Overstimulated

"Say what? You want me to nap, with all this excitement?"

Sometimes, even dedicated nappers get too overstimulated to sleep. If your sweetie just played "tickle my tummy" with her dad or had a shot of caffeine from your breast milk (or a piece of chocolate), she may have a hard time noticing that she's tuckered out.

And your swashbuckling little Christopher Columbus impersonator may fight napping because he's having so much fun exploring . . . he doesn't want to miss a thing.

So How Do You Switch Your Wide-Eyed Wrangler to Sleepy Mode?

Enjoy some fun quiet play with your child in his bedroom a couple of times a day. (Some kids resist going into their rooms because they know this means they'll have to stop playing and go to sleep.) That way, he won't only associate his room with "un-fun" naps.

Thirty minutes before naptime, engage in some quiet play and put on soft white noise in the background as a subconscious clue that sleep time is coming.

Then, for the nap, darken the room—as well as you can—and crank up a stronger rough, rumbly white noise—if your house is active, you may even need to start it a little louder than a shower. (Remember that whooshy fans, air filters, and wave sounds may totally fail because they're just too mild to really screen out disturbances.)

Napping Too Much? Or at the Wrong Time?

While too little naptime sleep is the biggest complaint I hear, some kids actually sleep too long during the day . . . and others sleep at oddball hours that don't work with their parents' schedules.

Typically, kids snooze one or two hours at each naptime. If your child is napping longer but still sleeping well at night, congratulations! You've hit the parent jackpot. But more often, kids who nap a lot end up needing a later bedtime . . . or waking more often at night. That's fine if it suits your life schedule—but if you'd like to shift some of that day sleep to the nighttime, it's pretty easy to do.

For example, say your child naps a lot and her bedtime is 8 P.M., but she's awake and chatty then and never falls asleep before 9:30. Try shortening her afternoon nap by fifteen minutes (so she's a bit more tired at night) and starting her bedtime routine at 9 P.M. Then, if that goes well, shorten her nap again and slide bedtime another fifteen minutes earlier. That should nestle her into the schedule you want. (You'll know you're shrinking her nap too much if she gets cranky in the early evening.)

How Temperament Can Trip Up Napping

Easy kids usually take things in stride: late naps, short naps, naps on the go. But other kids are not always . . . well, easy.

Sensitive kids need their naps to be just so. They may resist naps at the wrong time, in the wrong place (a neighbor's house, in the car), or with the wrong cues (without their special sheets, dollies, and sound).

Passionate, spirited kids often resist naps because they're having too much fun. If that sounds like your little guy, give him a gradual transition from play to pillow. Offer him a warning that sleep time is coming—for instance, say, "Naptime in three minutes!" or "Wow, you're really having fun playing. But do you remember what we're going to do when the dinger rings in five minutes? Right! It's naptime."

Don't Forget Your Trusty Sleep Cues!

What works at nighttime works in the daytime, too . . . so remember to use *all* the sleep cues we've talked about.

Nighttime white noise is like a young child's *teddy bear* of sound. But since daytime noises and distractions are usually quite a bit *louder* than nighttime disruptions, naptime noise should also be cranked up a notch. Expect to play it a little louder (the intensity of a shower) and use a sound that is a little rougher (like a hair dryer sound) than you do at night.

A mobile app, MP3 player, or portable CD lets you take this soothing sound anywhere. When your little Einstein hears the white noise, he'll remember, *Ahh, this sound means it's sleep time.*

And feel free to be creative as well. One mom told me she used an electric toothbrush to promote naps as she pushed the stroller around the neighborhood during walks!

Loveys (like pacifiers or blankies, and small stuffed animals) can also help naps. Make sure stuffed toys have no button eyes or removable parts that might cause choking or get stuck up the nose.

And don't forget other great cues, like lullabies, curtains to darken the room, a drop of lavender on the mattress or bed frame, and a little massage. These cues are especially handy when you're away from home.

Extra Tricks to Promote Naps

Another great napping tool is *twinkle interruptus* (see page 255).

For instance, if your angel tries to delay naptime by asking you for more stories, tuck him in and say, "Okay—let's read a story." Then pause partway through the book and do the "Wait! Wait! One second! I'll be right back" routine and leave the room. Return in ten seconds and continue the story. Gradually increase your time away, and eventually he will likely doze off before you return.

(Make sure you've first practiced *patience-stretching* a few times a day for a week, and you're using a rumbly white noise.)

Also, when your sweetie lies down, do a little *bedtime sweet talk*. Count and discuss any hand checks he has. Recall some of the good things that happened already that day. You might even *gossip* to his stuffed animals about how well he tried to do some new task.

When you're talking with him or his toys, remember to use the routine of a lullaby or work in cue words that he'll associate with naptime. For instance, say, "Let's tuck your puppy in for *sleepy-time* . . . let's tuck Patty Pig in for *sleepy-time* . . . they're so happy snuggling up at *sleepy-time*."

Finally, don't forget it's always preferable for your tyke to be a tiny bit awake when you place him in bed, so he can practice his self-soothing skills.

Common Questions About Naps

Q: My four-month-old only naps for thirty minutes. How can I make him nap longer?

Your curious little child probably doesn't want to miss any of the fun activities of the day! To encourage him to snooze longer, keep the room a little cool and reduce distractions (for example, turn off the phone). Certainly use a lovey and rough white noise (as loud as a shower). And, if he is a motion-loving baby who gets soothed with jiggling, rocking, and dancing, try letting him take his nap in the swing—*fully reclined,* swaddled, buckled in, on the fast speed. (Please take a look at pages 78–79 for a reminder of all the important swing safety steps.)

Also, make sure he's not getting any stimulants, like chocolate or caffeine-containing drinks.

Q: Are catnaps as good as regular naps?

Catnaps are great . . . for cats!

Okay, I admit it: some kids do just fine with a few fifteen-minute chunks of sleep in the car seat while mom or dad runs errands. But for many toddlers, it's just not enough. For these little ones, catnaps lead to cranky, moody behavior.

Catnaps often don't give kids the deep sleep they really need to feel rested and restored. Think of catnaps as like giving a run-down wind-up doll a couple of cranks of the key. It gets kids active again, but they run down and stop in just a few minutes!

This pattern can be pretty easy to change. Just push the first catnap off a little (avoiding the car or stroller or whatever place usually lulls your child to sleep). Make sure you're home at naptime so that when your child is sleepier, he can get a one- or two-hour nap.

Q: What should I do if my baby misses a nap?

First of all, don't worry if this happens occasionally. Kids miss naps all the time. Sometimes it's because there's so much going on in the house that they just blow right past the naptime. Other times, it's because they're starting to outgrow naps and skipping them every day or two.

If your sweetie misses a nap, you'll have to make a judgment call. In general, it's best if you can wait for the second naptime, but start it thirty to sixty minutes earlier. But if your child is so tired that he's getting cranky or bumping into walls, it's time for a power nap. In that case, it may make sense to have an early dinner and move bedtime a bit earlier for that one night.

Q: Is it okay for my child to nap in the playpen?

Sure. Just don't use it for discipline, too, or you'll jinx it by making it feel less like a sanctuary to treasure than a prison to avoid.

Q: My fifteen-month-old really fights his afternoon nap. Should I just put him down and let him "cry it out"?

CIO is pretty tough to use for naps because really tenacious kids are able to keep up their crying for thirty to sixty minutes. By then, the nap is over, everybody is cranky, and the rest of the day is miserable.

So even if you've opted for CIO at night, I would steer clear of it for naps. Once your child masters night sleeping, his day sleeping will probably spontaneously clear itself up. But if not, I suggest using the *twinkle interruptus* method of sleep training (see page 255). It's much easier on everyone in the family.

Q: Should I try to make my house totally silent at naptime?

Fact: Some parents tiptoe around for hours during naptime, terrified that an errant giggle or sneeze will rouse their little angel from sleep. But in reality, babies and toddlers find normal household noises soothing.

However, do set your phone on vibrate, because a shrill noise like a ringing phone can startle a snoozing baby or toddler. And be sure to keep the white noise going, because it can ease your little one back to sleep after the doorbell rings or the dog barks.

Rather than worrying too much about noise, think about light. Usually it's not necessary to have the room totally dark. However, some kids are very light-sensitive and have trouble sleeping when light is streaming through the curtains.

If you think this might be the case for your sweetie, buy heavy drapes that will keep most light out—or just use a big piece of heavy cardboard or a black-painted piece of Plexiglas to cover the window.

Q: I hate putting my toddler to bed when he's alert and having fun. Is it okay to delay naptime until he's sleepy?

I've talked about this in relation to sleep at night, and it's the same for daytime: don't wait until your darling "looks sleepy." He'll sleep longer and feel happier if he's in bed *before* he gets overtired. So if you're seeing yawning and eye-rubbing, you've already missed the boat a little.

Q: Would skipping the afternoon nap help my eighteen-month-old sleep better at night?

To know for sure how skipping naptime will affect your little friend, notice what happens the next time she slides through a whole day without napping. Most likely, she'll be fussing at dinner and become tearful or explosive at bedtime.

Parent educator Elizabeth Pantley calls this the "Volcano Effect" because your little one's stress builds and builds until she just goes blooey. It's not a pretty thing, and it shows you why those stress-busting naps are so crucial!

Crib Notes:
Reviewing *The Happiest Baby/ Toddler* Way

- For the first four months, babies benefit from swaddling and white noise for all naps. And some motion-loving babies even need to sleep in the swing (with your doctor's permission).

- To promote your baby's self-soothing skill, always place her down awake. If she has fallen asleep in your arms, jostle her awake when you slip her into the bassinet (the *wake-and-sleep* technique).

- Since daytime noises are often *louder* than nighttime disruptions, your infant will probably need a louder, rougher sound (as loud as a shower, as rough as a hair dryer) than he needs at night.

- White noise also promotes successful naps throughout the toddler years (including at day care).

- If your toddler resists napping, white noise, *patience-stretching,* and *twinkle interruptus* can help recapture his cooperation.

## CHAPTER FIFTEEN

Red Alerts and Special Situations

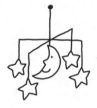

KEY POINTS:

★ **From asthma to seizures, medical problems can keep your child awake. Luckily, there are steps you can take to keep these sleep thieves from ruining your night.**

★ **Snoring may sound cute, but it's often a symptom of sleep-disordered breathing (SDB)—a common, sometimes serious, but *very* treatable problem.**

★ **Special situations like vacation trips can fracture your child's sleep—but there are some good ways to get it back on track.**

- ★ **The last thing you'll want to use to solve a sleep problem is medication. If your doctor is considering it, ask about using melatonin instead.**
- ★ **There are many ways to reduce *your* insomnia, so you can go from counting sheep to catching zzzz's.**

Each difficult moment has the potential to open my eyes and open my heart.

—MYLA KABAT-ZINN

When the Unexpected Happens . . . It's Your Time to Shine as a Parent

In the months before our babies arrive, we dream about the joys of parenting—rocking a cuddly baby, roughhousing with a tot, or taping finger paintings to the front of the fridge.

But we soon discover that along with these joys come many challenges. And when our young children need us the most, we learn just how strong we are.

But to be at our best, we need our kids to sleep . . . so we can, too.

In this chapter, I'll take a look at some medical issues that steal sleep—from vacation travel to asthma and snoring. In addition, I'll talk about ways to reduce the sleep challenges of autism and attention-deficit/hyperactivity disorder (ADHD), and what to do if *you* are battling insomnia.

Red Alerts—Medical Issues That Can Keep Your Child Awake

In earlier chapters, I discussed colds, the flu, and some other common sleep disruptors. Here are some additional medical problems that can cut down on slumber (and, in some cases, may even scare the heck out of you). The good news is that they're all treatable.

Nighttime Coughs—Allergies, Asthma, and Acid Reflux

Coughs typically get worse after lights-out. That's when croup kicks up spasms of coughing and when colds, sinusitis, and allergies cause mucus to drip down the back of the nose and throat, causing a wet, gunk-filled cough. Night cough can also be a sign of asthma (either dry, wheezy coughs or thick, wet, chesty rumbles) or an irritation from acid reflux. Here's a look at each problem.

Allergies, Colds, and Sinus Infections

All kids get nose colds, 40 percent experience allergies, and many get occasional sinusitis. I'm lumping them all together because they all have one thing in common: they trigger a loose nighttime cough caused by mucus meandering down the back of the throat (postnasal drip).

Clear, drippy colds can strike your child every other month during the toddler years. (You'll find strategies for handling colds on page 108.) Sinus infections, on the other hand, cause dark circles under the eyes, green or yellow nose goop, fever, and low energy. These clearly require your doctor's attention.

Allergies also cause clear, drippy noses (with some sneezing, coughing, and nose itching), but they tend to go on and on and often require a doctor's attention to diagnose and treat. So if your child's night cough continues for weeks, consider that it may be caused by allergies.

While some kids are allergic to foods (like dairy or wheat), airborne allergens are much more common. The chief culprits include:

- **Dust (in the mattress, blanket, pillow, or carpeting)**
- **Mildew in the walls or closet**
- **Smoke from cigarettes, fireplaces, candles, or wood-burning stoves**
- **Fumes from fresh paint, new carpet, air fresheners, or particleboard furniture**
- **Outdoor pollen**

When you discuss this issue with your child's health-care provider, he or she may suggest simple steps like these to start:

1. **CLEAR THE AIR. Open the window and ventilate the room every day. Put clean filters in your heat vents and air-conditioning air intake. Wash your carpet or rug, remove or wash stuffed animals, replace feather pillows and blankets with hypoallergenic fibers, and get special allergy-proof coverings for your child's mattress and pillow. Ask your doctor about using a HEPA (*high-efficiency particulate air*) filter in the room or a dehumidifier in a musty, dank closet or basement. (Many insurance companies will pay for these if you have a doctor's prescription.)**

2. **BAN SMOKING. Smoking does terrible things to everyone in the family, triggering everything from colds and sinus infections to emphysema . . . and cancer! And it's not okay to smoke in your home even when your child isn't there. Smoke clings to the walls and drapes for hours and hours.**

3. **STOP THE DRIP. As I've mentioned, when your child lies down, mucus from a runny nose can drip down the back of the throat and trigger coughing or wheezing. Ask your doctor about ways to stop an allergic drip. Options include oral antihistamines; medicated nasal spray (steroid, decongestant, or mast cell stabilizer); environmental changes; elimination diets; and allergy shots.**

Asthma—the Night Cough That Can Get Much Worse

Tiny muscle threads open and close the breathing tubes deep in the chest. In asthma, these muscles tighten too much, either all at once (an asthma attack) or bit by bit.

If the blockage is less than 50 percent, there are usually no symptoms whatsoever. A tightening greater than 50 percent causes a dry night cough. And, as the tubes get even tighter, children start to sense a tight feeling in the chest, then develop a wet cough, and finally start making a high-pitched wheezy sound, primarily when breathing out.

During the tight spasms of an asthma attack, each exhalation gets longer and more labored. Your child may flare his nostrils and suck in air so hard that the skin in the little notch at the top of the breastbone gets visibly pulled in with every breath.

Asthma is more common at night, especially if a child's bedroom is dusty or his bedding contains allergens like feathers or invisible dust mites.

Usually, I'm pretty conservative and try to treat ailments without medicine, but I am fast to use medication when I suspect asthma. I like to nip it in the bud—during early coughing—rather than waiting for a child's lungs to get so tight that he wheezes. (And be sure you always take the medicine with you on trips and vacations.)

BTW, although a possible side effect of asthma medication is restlessness, it usually ends up *boosting* sleep by reducing the spasms of cough and the agitation caused by difficult breathing.

Inhaled Objects: Night Coughs That Require Immediate Surgery

Jeanette was telling her pediatrician about eighteen-month-old Suri's nightly cough when she suddenly remembered that Suri had been playing in a little fireplace a few weeks earlier when she suddenly experienced a coughing fit.

This prompted her alert doctor to investigate whether Suri might have inhaled something during her little adventure. And indeed, she had: a small piece of plastic. Suri needed surgery to remove the object.

If your child's coughing comes on suddenly and doesn't get better despite everything you do, ask your pediatrician if the culprit might be a nut, a piece of plastic, gravel, or some other object that went down "the wrong pipe."

The Burning Night Cough of Acid Reflux

I talked earlier about acid reflux (also called gastroesophageal reflux disease, or GERD), but here's a quick review.

Most babies have a little bit of acid reflux; we just call it "spitting up." It peaks at four months of age and is usually gone by one year. While it rarely causes crying or colic, it can definitely cause breathing problems like nighttime cough, hoarseness, and wheezing. This happens when the stomach juices sneak up into the throat and then down into the lungs, irritating everything they touch.

If your child has a persistent cough, ask your doctor if reflux might be the cause. The solution may involve adding a little rice to thicken your child's formula, changing her sleeping position, eliminating cow's milk products, or giving her medication.

Sleep-Disordered Breathing: Kids Who Snore and Choke

Carol's sweet little three-year-old, Timmy, developed cold after cold shortly after starting preschool. But that wasn't the worst of it! He also became increasingly crabby, a superpicky eater, and openly defiant, fighting and screaming each morning at preschool drop-off.

Carol's mother-in-law accused her of spoiling Timmy ("Your little boy needs some good, old-fashioned discipline"). But Carol's mommy instincts told her it was something else, and she decided to have her son evaluated.

Among her litany of questions, the doctor asked if Timmy was snoring. "Like a sailor," laughed Carol. The doctor then asked if

Timmy woke up with drool on his pillow and dark circles under his eyes. "Every morning," Carol said with a look of surprise.

Bingo! As soon as the doctor had Timmy open and say "Ahhhh," she turned to Carol and said, "Wow! His tonsils are huge! No wonder he's having problems—he's probably choking all night long."

The doctor said that Timmy had sleep apnea and scheduled him to have his tonsils and adenoids removed. Carol felt terrible that Timmy had suffered for so long, but she also felt relieved to find a clear—and fixable—cause of his problems.

"It was a miracle!" she proclaimed, a week after the surgery. "He's eating great, gaining weight, and sleeping superbly. In fact, he's now so quiet at night I have to get close to his face just to make sure he's breathing."

A child with sleep-disordered breathing (SBD) struggles to inhale enough air while he's asleep. It gets worse when the child lies on his back (because gravity causes the throat to narrow even more), and a tot with SDB may often arch his neck and open his mouth in an attempt to get as much air in as possible.

SBD can start as early as two years of age—when the tonsils and adenoids are growing fast—and go all the way through the teen years and adulthood.

What Are Tonsils and Adenoids?

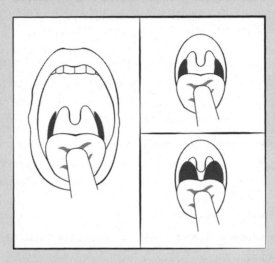

Tonsils and adenoids are special lymph glands that serve as our own personal Homeland Security squad, constantly oozing out antibodies and directing white blood cells to capture viruses and germs before they can sneak into the body. (Shown here in black.)

These big lumps usually don't cause problems during the day. But during sleep, when the throat muscles relax and sag, large tonsils and adenoids can cause the whole tunnel to narrow dramatically. That makes a child's throat collapse with each breath, like a paper bag caving in when you suck the air out of it.

About 7 to 12 percent of young children have primary snoring (more than three times a week) caused by mild air blockage. But 1 to 3 percent of children develop severe blockage (90–100 percent) and experience *apnea*.

Obstructive sleep apnea, or OSA, is sleep-disordered breathing that gets so bad the throat closes completely and the child goes more than ten seconds with absolutely no breathing. This can seem quite scary, but *don't panic*! If your child's breathing stops for too long, he'll automatically wake up and start breathing again.

Kids with SBD may startle awake with a snort or gasp dozens or *hundreds* of times each night! No wonder kids like Timmy yawn all day and get irritable, defiant, "hyper," forgetful, and accident-prone. SBD also weakens the immune system, undermines learning, and can lead to high blood pressure and heart strain.

Do you think your child might have SBD? Check with your doctor if he:

- **Sleeps with his mouth open**
- **Snores or wakes with a loud snort**
- **Has a nasal, gravelly voice**
- **Drools on the pillowcase**
- **Breathes through his mouth instead of his nose**
- **Has morning headaches**
- **Resists swallowing food because it "scratches" on the way down**
- **Is excessively sleepy**

Obesity and SDB . . . a Vicious Cycle

Like Timmy, many kids with Sleep Disordered Breathing are rail thin because they just have no appetite. However, many other kids with this problem are quite overweight.

It is obvious that obese children have layers of fat right under their skin. But what we can't see is that they also have thin ripples of fat deposited under the wet membranes at the back of the nose and throat. This fat can create a blockage, making it hard to breathe when a child is lying on the back.

This obstruction—on top of the blockage from big tonsils and adenoids—can keep a child from getting restful sleep. And that's a big problem because poor sleep can lead to even more weight gain as kids:

- Get less exercise (because they're tired)

- Eat more (because fatigue makes them crave fats and sugar and lowers their impulse control . . . and they're watching more TV and being tempted by all the junk food commercials)

- Develop insulin resistance, causing increased obesity and raising the risk of diabetes

A Few Simple Ideas to Help a Child with SDB Rest Easier

If your child snores or has other symptoms of SDB, opening up his throat a little bit more can make a huge difference. So, while you're waiting for your doctor to finish her evaluation, try these simple steps:

- Elevate the head of the mattress by putting a folded towel or blanket under it.

- Moisturize the air with a cool mist humidifier. (Clean it thoroughly to avoid mold. See page 267.)

- Take your child off dairy products (milk, cheese, etc.) for two weeks.

- Have her tested for allergies. (If the doctor confirms this problem, follow the steps on page 320.)

- Ask your doctor about a trial of medication to shrink the tonsils (like an oral or inhaled corticosteroid or a leukotriene inhibitor).

- Keep pets out of your child's bedroom.

If the snoring and other sleep problems don't get better after a week or two, then your child's doctor may recommend removing her tonsils and/or adenoids.

The Return of the T&A

If your child has SBD and initial treatments aren't working, your health-care provider may recommend an operation called *T&A surgery* to remove the tonsils and adenoids.

After World War II, doctors performed T&A surgery at the drop of a hat. In the 1970s, we radically reduced the number of kids getting this surgery. But in the 1990s, we began to realize that the operation was a *huge* help for children with blocked breathing.

T&A surgery is currently the second-most-common outpatient operation for children. And thankfully, it resolves SBD symptoms in 70 to 90 percent of uncomplicated cases.

But here's one caution: if your child is overweight or older than seven years of age, get a second opinion before agreeing to T&A surgery. Kids in these categories tend to have less success with the procedure. In fact, 50 percent of obese children can have residual symptoms after a T&A.

Nighttime Seizures

A seizure (also called a convulsion) occurs when the brain short-circuits. This can cause uncontrolled body jerks, an inability to communicate, and urination.

Night is actually a common time for seizures. The brain is more susceptible to these electrical eruptions when it's overly tired and just entering sleep . . . or just awaking.

It's easy to mistake the screaming and unresponsiveness of a night terror for a seizure. But while night terrors terrorize *us*, they lack the cardinal signs of seizures: drooling, limb twitching, tongue biting, and incontinence.

Night seizures may be triggered by a sudden surge of fever. It's pretty clear when this is the case because a child usually is flushed red and hot to the touch.

But when there's no obvious reason for a night seizure, the cause may be *benign rolandic epilepsy* (also called *benign focal epilepsy of childhood*).

This problem can start as early as three years of age, although it usually doesn't begin before kids are five. These seizures are often overlooked for a long time because they happen during sleep. But once the diagnosis is suspected, parents often report that their kids have been sleeping less, exhausted during the day, and experiencing night terrors and sleepwalking for weeks or months. Fortunately, the seizures cause absolutely no serious health problems and disappear by the teen years.

The diagnosis of seizures requires a full medical evaluation, including a sleep EEG (electroencephalogram) to record the electrical activity in the brain (although sometimes the EEG may be normal). Many children don't need any treatment at all, while others benefit from taking an anticonvulsant drug.

Autism and Other Developmental Problems

Approximately 1 percent of all children born in the United States each year are diagnosed with autism. Children on the autistic spectrum frequently have problems with sleep.

Interestingly, these children often instinctively use some of the 5 S's to calm themselves! They hum, spin, and make repetitive motions. And many teachers and parents notice that they calm faster with rocking, white noise, and the use of heavy blankets.

If your child has autism spectrum disorder (ASD) and trouble sleeping, you may be surprised to learn that research reveals that—on average—children on the autism spectrum sleep only *a bit* less than typically developing kids. However, caring for these kids can be so exhausting that it makes even normal sleep disruptions hard to handle.

If your child has autism and sleep difficulties, here are some things you can try to get slumber back into your life:

Prepare for success. Reduce junk food (candy, chips, fried food, sweet breakfast cereal, and sugary drinks—including undiluted apple juice—and anything with caffeine, including chocolate, teas, herbs, and supplements). Ask your pediatrician about the potential benefits of a gluten-free, casein-free diet. (Some parents of children with autism find this diet works wonders.) Also, make sure your child gets plenty of sunshine, fresh air, and exercise during the day.

In the evening, you'll want to use *every* trick in your bedtime routine. An hour before sleepy-time, dim the lights, turn off the TV, stop roughhousing, *and* turn on some soft white noise in the background. Children on the autism spectrum can be especially rigid and resistant to change, so make sure you follow your beddy-bye ritual to the letter.

Create good nighttime habits. If your child's nightly cries disturb the family or neighbors, you might be tempted to sleep with him to keep him calm. But if you can place your child in bed awake, he's more likely to learn to self-soothe and put himself back to sleep if he wakes during the night.

To boost your chances of success, use the rough, rumbly white noise CD or app all night long.

If you haven't been using white noise, introduce it slowly. Initially, play it quietly in the background during the evening (some kids do well with it during the day, too). Next, begin using it quietly all night long. Gradually increase the volume over three or four nights until it reaches the noise level of a shower.

Many parents find that the *right-brain Happiest Toddler* communication tips (like *Toddler-ese, gossiping, magic breathing,* and *patience-*

stretching described on pages 212–16) are particularly helpful with children with *left-brain* verbal delays (like autism) throughout childhood . . . and well beyond.

Other calming sleep routines to consider include:

- **Putting your child in a heavy vest or using a heavy blanket.**

- **Brushing your child's skin gently with a hairbrush or backscratcher.**

- **Snuggly swaddling his upper body.**

- **Using a very silky blanket as a comforting lovey.**

- **Spraying a little lavender mist into the air as a signal that it's time to sleep.**

- **Dimming or blocking all lights (including the TV, clocks, hall lights under the door, and streetlights outside the window). One exception: a very dim night-light may reduce your child's anxiety.**

Very delayed children may require *fortified* cribs (with safety netting and higher side rails) or alarms on the door to keep them from leaving the bedroom and disrupting the whole family's sleep.

Finally, your doctor may also recommend giving a magnesium supplement; or 3–10 mg of over-the-counter melatonin thirty minutes before bedtime; or perhaps even a prescription sleep medicine.

ADHD—Hyperactivity Makes Sleeping Hard

Attention-deficit/hyperactivity disorder (ADHD) is a neurodevelopmental disorder said to affect about 5 percent of children (and adults).

Kids with ADHD are often *hyper,* forgetful, impulsive, and distractible. (Of course, these can all be normal behaviors for any toddler, which is why doctors are *very hesitant* to diagnose ADHD before the age of five.)

Short sleep and hyperactivity spiral together. Children with ADHD tend to get especially defiant, moody, and wild when they're tired. Unfortunately, that usually results in less sleep and kids who act even *more* wired the next day . . . and so the cycle continues.

The ADHD–Poor Sleep Relationship

Children with ADHD often have sleep problems. But can poor sleep actually *trigger* some kids' hyperactivity?

A study of nearly seven thousand California kids showed that preschoolers who slept less were rated by their parents as more hyperactive and less attentive in kindergarten.

The lead researcher, Erika Gaylor, speculated that poor sleep may push some children toward being more impulsive and inattentive later in life.

This suspicion that poor early sleep may lead to ADHD later in childhood is supported by a Canadian study. Researchers studying more than a thousand children (two to six years old) found that *toddlers* sleeping less than ten hours a night were twice as likely to become hyperactive—later, when they became *preschoolers*!

Sleep problems are very common in ADHD. These problems may be related to the ADHD itself or to co-occurring problems like anxiety or fear.

Also, one common effect of ADHD medicines in young children is poor sleep. (Many ADHD medications are stimulants, chemically related to amphetamine.)

If your child is diagnosed with ADHD, here are the best ways to promote sleep:

- Make sure your child exercises daily and gets some sun every day.

- Give regular, healthy meals high in fiber and containing protein and vegetables.

- Avoid foods with artificial colors and flavors.

- Avoid sweetened breakfast cereals and sugary drinks, including undiluted juice. Instead, offer naturally sweet mint or chamomile tea. (Interestingly, caffeinated drinks have been used for decades to *reduce* the wild behavior and impulsivity of ADHD.)

- Keep your nap schedule consistent.

- Practice *magic breathing* and *patience-stretching* every day.

- Create stable and reliable prebedtime routines, including quiet play, reading, massage, white noise, and dimmed lights. (Turn off bright TV, computer, and video game screens.)

- Take the TV out of his room.

- Avoid roughhousing, family arguments, and loud or scary TV shows before bedtime.

- Get your child into bed *before* he's overtired.

- Ask your child's doctor about medication side effects and see if you use a regimen that minimizes sleep problems. (Also, ask about using melatonin as a sleep enhancer.)

- Treat any allergies, snoring problems, or other sleep disruptors.

Do Kids Ever Need Sleeping Pills?

In generations past, parents often gave small children "a little something" to put them to sleep—from a few drops of opium to a nip of brandy. These days, parents are more likely to ask for a prescription.

However, when it comes to giving medicine to young children, the best rule of thumb is *less is better*. This is especially true for sleep medications. These can be too strong or backfire and accidentally make kids hyper! In fact, none of the common adult sleep medicines are approved by the Food and Drug Administration (FDA) for use in children.

However, one supplement that's been shown to occasionally help children with serious sleep problems is melatonin. As you'll remember, our brains make melatonin every evening as the lights dim, but this hormone is also available as an over-the-counter supplement.

A standard toddler dose is 1 mg, given an hour before bedtime. Higher doses (3–10 mg) have been shown to help kids with medically related sleep difficulties such as blindness, autism, or ADHD.

Like any medication, melatonin can have side effects. These may include daytime grogginess, headache, and very vivid dreams.

Even though the medicine is readily available, *always* consult your doctor before using it. And only use a very reputable brand of melatonin. The FDA doesn't regulate the supplements, so their purity is not assured. Also, avoid melatonin that was harvested from the brains of animals.

Insomnia—When *You* Can't Sleep

Dr. Kathryn Sharkey, a sleep expert from Brown University, told the *New York Times*, "A female patient will come in complaining of insomnia, and when asked how long she's had it, will say, 'Fifteen years—ever since my baby was born.'"

Almost everyone suffers from sleep deprivation at some point in life. But it can be so bad when you have a young child that it can literally feel like torture. Worse, as exhaustion builds, you may get so anxious—"I have to fall asleep before the baby wakes again!"—that it's even *harder* to fall asleep.

Sure, you're focused on giving your baby lots of care and love.

But that shouldn't be at the expense of your health. In fact, if your baby could speak, he'd say, "Hey—I need you a lot, so stay healthy!"

If you're getting your baby's sleep under control but battling insomnia yourself, try these sleep-enhancing tips.

1. Prepare Your Room

Make sure your room is a little cool, with good ventilation.

And remember that white noise isn't just for your baby! The brain has a hard time paying attention to two things at once, so white noise covers over disturbing sounds from the next-door neighbors or passing trucks or trains. Try white noise for yourself (start it softly, an hour before sleep to give your brain a few days to get used to it).

Even better, white noise covers over the flood of worries that may be preventing sleep from coming. These sounds allow your tired brain to ignore burdensome thoughts and slide more easily into sleep. Many moms and dads find a *rain on the roof* sound soothing; just start it softly, about an hour before bedtime, and increase the nighttime volume over time.

Note: Not all white noise is the same. *Higher-pitched sounds can be alerting, rather than calming.* So, if you find white noise annoying, try a lower-pitched sound; for example, the specially engineered *Happiest Baby* white noise tracks.

And here's another idea: keep a pen and paper by your bed so you can just jot down important ideas, rather than staying up and fretting that you might forget them.

Most important of all, remember: light is the enemy of sleep! For thousands of years, darkness was the brain's cue to get ready to sleep. (Electric lights have only been around for a hundred years.)

Your house lights trick your brain into thinking it's still afternoon. The brain then shuts off your natural melatonin, which delays your drowsiness until much later at night. You'll feel more alert in the evening, but you'll be exhausted when your little one wakes you up at the crack of dawn.

So an hour before bedtime, dim the lights . . . and dim or turn off your computer or cell-phone screen, too! While you sleep, wear an eye mask or put a towel over any bright lights in your bedroom (cable boxes, alarm clocks, etc.).

When you wake up in the middle of the night, *don't turn on the lights.* Use a little flashlight or night-light, and resist the urge to look at the bright screen of your cell phone to check your e-mails or texts.

2. Prepare Your Body

Get some sunshine every day to set your internal clock. If you live somewhere with a long, dark winter, consider getting special SAD lights (for the prevention of seasonal affective disorder).

No matter how hectic your schedule is, get some exercise every day. Aim for at least twenty minutes (thirty is even better)—but in a pinch, go out for one or two laps around the block. If you can, get a friend to go with you. It's usually best not to exercise within three hours of bedtime.

A little daytime nap can be a big help, too.

And at the risk of sounding like your mother . . . are you eating well? Exhaustion can make you eat impulsively, cause you to crave carbs and fat, and throw your metabolism into a weight-gaining spiral. Weight gain, in turn, can lead to poor sleep . . . which can start a vicious cycle.

Nip that cycle in the bud by eating three medium meals a day and a snack or two. Choose whole grains or high-fiber foods and snack on fruits, veggies, hummus, and crackers. Try to skip the Twinkies and reach for foods with some protein, like nuts, trail mix, a fried egg, or a glass of warm milk (maybe with some honey).

Make lunch your big meal and eat dinner at least three hours before bedtime. And avoid anything with caffeine, including coffee, tea, cola, chocolate, and energy drinks. Decongestants, diet supplements, and Chinese herbs can also contain stimulants that thwart sleep.

Some warm mint tea is soothing and can put you in the mood for slumber, too. (In Serbian, mint is called *nana*—which means "grandma"—because it's what Grandma offers to comfort her family.)

If your partner snores, a strong white noise may reduce your brain's attention to the ruckus. Also, try the same strategies on him that I've talked about for preventing snoring in kids (see page 326). And get that snoring checked out, because it might be a sign of a correctable problem.

3. Prepare Your Mind

Laughter is one of the world's best stress reducers. So dig out your favorite funny movies, read a book that makes you giggle, or call a friend with a great sense of humor.

When you lie down, do a little *bedtime sweet talk* with *yourself*. And I know I'm sounding like your mother again . . . but count your blessings several times each day. Each time, fill your heart with gratitude and love.

Also, don't sweat the small stuff. Turn off your phone, delay writing your thank-you notes, and put off chores like vacuuming.

Avoid sleeping medications, but ask your doctor about taking some magnesium, valerian, or melatonin. These may promote sleep without making you too drowsy to respond to your child's middle-of-the-night needs. Resist the urge to have a beer or a glass of wine before bedtime; it's likely to lead to more nighttime waking, and it can reduce your ability to respond to your baby's needs. (And if you're nursing, remember that what you drink, your baby drinks.)

Finally, create a regular "wind-down" routine for yourself in the evening. Give your baby a massage (it'll relax both of you), listen to quiet music, turn off the TV, read a book, or write in a journal.

Meditation: Let Go of the Chaos to Help You Sleep Sweetly

I know it's hard for a hectic multitasker to suddenly turn into a Zen Buddhist at bedtime. But once your child is asleep, it's superimportant for you to be able to come in for a soft landing after a full and demanding day. One way to accomplish this is to practice some breathing/calming exercises.

Two key steps in this simple act are letting your face muscles fully relax—like a wet rag. Facial tension keeps you in stress, and a relaxed expression or even a hint of a smile gives your body the cue to relax. And really slow your breathing down, especially paying attention to making your breathing out as long and as slow as your breathing in. Deep breaths can have an instantaneous effect, releasing a wave of calm.

As you breathe in and out, let each breath fill your heart with happiness as you think about the things that bless you in your life or the activities you look forward to doing tomorrow.

Also, visualize a safe, cozy place. Imagine a warm day at the beach, or picture yourself simply lying on the couch all warm and comfy.

If you want some help getting started, visit UCLA's Mindfulness Awareness Research Center (MARC) website at http://marc.ucla .edu/.

The Hidden Blessings of Trying Times

From sniffles to sleep apnea, your little child may give you plenty of things to worry about in the early years. But it's during these small crises (or sometimes bigger ones) that you'll truly earn your stripes as a parent!

What's more, these trying times will strengthen the bonds between you and your child. Just as you earn your baby's trust in the early days by being there with warm milk and loving arms, you'll enhance your child's confidence with your loving attention and comforting routines during rocky times.

So when the skies occasionally cloud over, be there and be strong for your precious little child. Let her know that she can count on you to understand and to help, and she'll reward you many times over in the years to come with her love and trust.

Crib Notes:
Reviewing *The Happiest Baby* Way

- Autism or ADHD can interfere with your child's much-needed sleep (and yours)—but melatonin and white noise can help you both rest longer.

- An hour before sleep, dim the house lights, tune up the white noise, and turn off the TV—and any bright screen (like your computer or cell phone).

- At night, use an eye mask (to block any light coming in through the window) and *rain on the roof* white noise.

- If you are not used to white noise all night (or find it annoying), use a low-pitched type of sound and begin it—softly—one hour before sleep. Take a week to gradually increase the volume, until it is as loud as a soft shower.

- When you lie down, do a little *bedtime sweet talk*—with yourself—to count your blessings!

Appendix

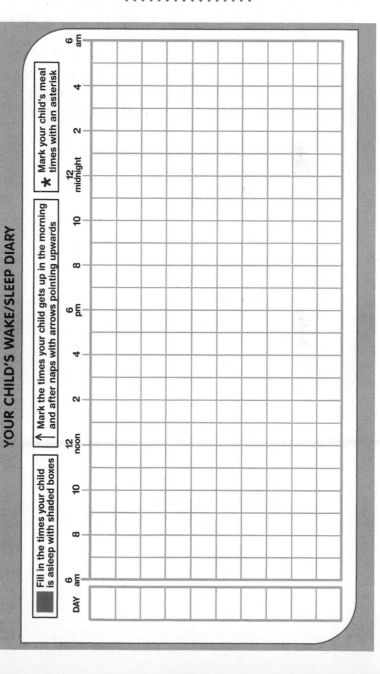

YOUR CHILD'S WAKE/SLEEP DIARY

Fill in the times your child is asleep with shaded boxes

↑ Mark the times your child gets up in the morning and after naps with arrows pointing upwards

★ Mark your child's meal times with an asterisk

DAY

6 am | 8 | 10 | 12 noon | 2 | 4 | 6 pm | 8 | 10 | 12 midnight | 2 | 4 | 6 am

Sample Sleep Schedules

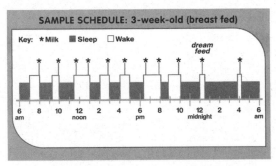

SAMPLE SCHEDULE: 3-week-old (breast fed)

Key: ★ Milk ■ Sleep ☐ Wake

dream feed

6 am 8 10 12 noon 2 4 6 pm 8 10 12 midnight 2 4 6 am

Daytime starts: 7 am
Night sleep starts: 10 pm
# of feeds/24 hrs: 9-12
# of naps/24 hrs: 3-6

Daytime sleep: 5-8 hrs
Longest night sleep: 3-5 hrs
Total night sleep: 7-8 hrs
Total sleep/24 hrs: 12-16 hrs

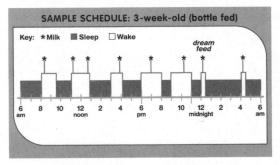

SAMPLE SCHEDULE: 3-week-old (bottle fed)

Key: ★ Milk ■ Sleep ☐ Wake

dream feed

6 am 8 10 12 noon 2 4 6 pm 8 10 12 midnight 2 4 6 am

Daytime starts: 7 am
Night sleep starts: 10 pm
# of feeds/24 hrs: 7-10
# of naps/24 hrs: 4-6

Daytime sleep: 5-8 hrs
Longest night sleep: 4-5 hrs
Total night sleep: 7-8 hrs
Total sleep/24 hrs: 12-16 hrs

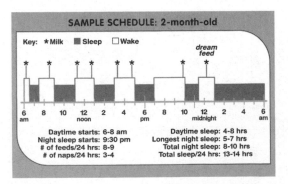

SAMPLE SCHEDULE: 2-month-old

Key: ★ Milk ■ Sleep ☐ Wake

dream feed

6 am 8 10 12 noon 2 4 6 pm 8 10 12 midnight 2 4 6 am

Daytime starts: 6-8 am
Night sleep starts: 9:30 pm
# of feeds/24 hrs: 8-9
# of naps/24 hrs: 3-4

Daytime sleep: 4-8 hrs
Longest night sleep: 5-7 hrs
Total night sleep: 8-10 hrs
Total sleep/24 hrs: 13-14 hrs

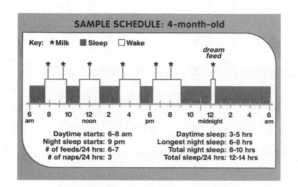

SAMPLE SCHEDULE: 4-month-old

Key: ★ Milk ■ Sleep □ Wake

dream feed

6 am 8 10 12 noon 2 4 6 pm 8 10 12 midnight 2 4 6 am

Daytime starts: 6-8 am
Night sleep starts: 9 pm
# of feeds/24 hrs: 6-7
# of naps/24 hrs: 3

Daytime sleep: 3-5 hrs
Longest night sleep: 6-8 hrs
Total night sleep: 8-10 hrs
Total sleep/24 hrs: 12-14 hrs

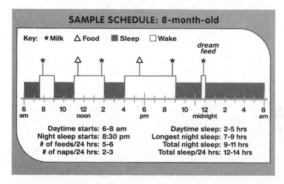

SAMPLE SCHEDULE: 8-month-old

Key: ★ Milk △ Food ■ Sleep □ Wake

dream feed

6 am 8 10 12 noon 2 4 6 pm 8 10 12 midnight 2 4 6 am

Daytime starts: 6-8 am
Night sleep starts: 8:30 pm
# of feeds/24 hrs: 5-6
# of naps/24 hrs: 2-3

Daytime sleep: 2-5 hrs
Longest night sleep: 7-9 hrs
Total night sleep: 9-11 hrs
Total sleep/24 hrs: 12-14 hrs

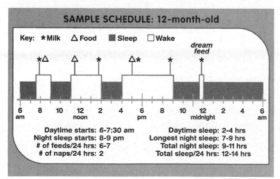

SAMPLE SCHEDULE: 12-month-old

Key: ★ Milk △ Food ■ Sleep □ Wake

dream feed

6 am 8 10 12 noon 2 4 6 pm 8 10 12 midnight 2 4 6 am

Daytime starts: 6-7:30 am
Night sleep starts: 8-9 pm
# of feeds/24 hrs: 6-7
# of naps/24 hrs: 2

Daytime sleep: 2-4 hrs
Longest night sleep: 7-9 hrs
Total night sleep: 9-11 hrs
Total sleep/24 hrs: 12-14 hrs

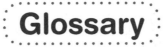

Glossary

The Happiest Baby and **The Happiest Toddler**
Key Terms and Sleep Solutions

Beddy-Bye book
A special book you make for your tot filled with pictures/photos/drawings and captions that narrate a typical day in your child's life (especially your evening and bedtime routines). Reviewing this together every day will make it easier for him to know exactly how to succeed at bedtime (page 240).

Bedtime sweet talk
A nightly routine where you snuggle together after tuck-in and remind your child of the many interesting experiences and good things she did that day (counting her hand checks and recalling why each one was given) and preview some of the fun things she can look forward to the next day (page 244).

Calming reflex
The automatic off-switch for crying and on-switch for sleep that all babies are born with (page 64).

Circadian rhythm
Our "inner clock" that tells us when to be awake and when to slumber peacefully. Bright light turns it on and off by coordinating the release of melatonin by the pineal gland (page 15).

Cluster feeds
Closely spaced feedings in the evening that can fill your child with calories to reduce the chance of waking in hunger during the night (page 168).

Dream feed
Waking your sleeping child up to give a night time snack of milk to reduce the chance of waking in hunger during the night (page 168).

Fairy tales
Little stories you make up to illustrate a specific lesson you want your child to learn (page 239).

Family meetings
A short parent-child meeting to discuss what he is doing well and what could be better. The goal is to agree on a way to encourage two to three specific good behaviors using a small reward or incentive (page 217).

Fast-Food Rule
When talking to anyone (adult or child) who is upset, before saying your reassurance, solution, or criticism, first say a couple of phrases acknowledging how she's feeling. This will help her calm down and be able to fully listen to your ideas (page 211).

Five S's
Five specific steps—swaddling, stomach or side, shushing, swinging, sucking—that turn on the *calming reflex* (soothing infant crying and boosting sleep in babies, infants, and toddlers (page 64).

Fourth trimester
The first three months of a baby's life (page 61).

Gossiping
A way to "supersize" the impact of your praise (or criticism) by letting your child overhear you whispering comments about his behavior to someone else . . . or even to a stuffed animal (page 215).

Hand checks
Little pen marks or ink stamps you put on the back of your child's hand to acknowledge and reward good deeds (page 215).

Longer-and-longer
A sleep-training approach where the infant is placed in bed and allowed to

cry, while the parents make increasingly less frequent visits to check her (every 5, 10, 15 minutes, etc.) (page 186).

Lovey
A cuddly "companion"—like a silky blanket or stuffed animal—which your toddler can snuggle with for comfort and reassurance. Also called a transitional object (page 150).

Magic breathing
Deep breathing that helps toddlers develop self-control and reduce stress (page 214).

Melatonin
A natural hormone (and an over-the-counter sleep supplement) that helps bring on sleep (page 135).

NREM sleep
Restful (non-dream) sleep. It comes in three increasingly restorative levels, from light to deep (page 18).

Patience-stretching
A way to increasingly prolong a child's ability to control her impulses and wait patiently (page 213).

Pick up/put down
A no-tears sleep-training method where you repeatedly pick your fussing child out of bed and then replace her once she calms (page 190).

Playing the boob
A fast way to boost confidence and reduce defiance by acting a bit slow and klutzy and thus allowing your tot to feel stronger, faster, and smarter than you (page 218).

Putting your child "on hold"
A method using *patience-stretching* to sidestep your child's whining and unreasonable demands (page 279).

REM sleep
Rapid eye movement sleep—when dreams occur and memories are built (page 18).

Reverse psychology
A clever way to get your tot to do something by suggesting that she *shouldn't* do it—for instance, by pulling gently on her pacifier rather than pushing it into her mouth (page 83).

Role-playing
Letting your child "act out" different roles in a little story you make up.

Have the characters practice good behaviors and overcome bad ones (pages 273–274).

Side-door lessons
Kids learn more from what they see others doing (or accidentally overhear) than from our sermons and instructions. I think of this type of indirect lesson—like fairy tales, role-playing, and *gossiping*—as learning . . . through the *side door* (page 238).

Sleep cues
Loveys, white noise, and other clues remind your tot that it's time to relax and fall asleep (page 61).

Sleep cycle
A segment of sleep made up of a roller-coaster-like flow from light to deep NREM sleep and then back up to light NREM sleep, followed by a short piece of REM sleep. This pattern repeats (cycles) over and over again through the night (page 18).

Special time
A fun daily routine where you show your child how important she is to you by giving her one or two short sessions (five to ten minutes) of your uninterrupted attention and play (page 209).

Star charts
A tool for improving an older toddler's cooperation by rewarding your child for accomplishing a few specific behaviors with little stars (or stickers) placed onto a daily chart (page 215).

State control
Your tot's ability to stay alert, stay asleep, and self-calm . . . even after an upsetting experience (page 34).

Temperament
Your child's personality—calm, sensitive, or spirited. It's a big factor in how she behaves and how she sleeps (page 33).

Twinkle interruptus
My favorite no-cry style of sleep training! This method uses white noise and training your toddler in *patience-stretching* to help him learn how to fall asleep on his own (page 255).

Wake and sleep
Teach infants to self-soothe in the middle of the night by putting them into bed at least a little awake. So, infants who fall asleep in your arms should be roused—a bit—when placed in the crib and then allowed to doze off on their own (page 88).

White noise
Rumbly, whooshy noise that imitates the sound of the womb, turns on the *calming reflex* during the early months, and acts as a powerful sleep cue for older infants and toddlers—and even adults (page 71).

Win-win solutions
No one likes to lose. When you have conflicts with your toddler, teach him the art of compromise by seeking out solutions where he gets some of what he wants and you do, too (page 248).

References

The following is a listing of many of the studies cited in this book.

Chapter 1

Anders TF, and Keener MA. Developmental courses of night-time sleep-wake patterns in full-term and premature infants during the first year of life I. *Sleep* 1985; 8: 173–92.

Aserinsky E, and Kleitman N. Regularly occurring periods of eye mobility and concomitant phenomena during sleep. *Science* 1953; 18: 273–74.

Axelsson J, et al. Beauty sleep: experimental study on the perceived health and attractiveness of sleep deprived people. *BMJ* 2010; 341:6614.

Christensen H, et al. Cognition in pregnancy and motherhood: prospective cohort study. *British Journal of Psychiatry* 2010; 196: 126–32.

Drosopoulos S, et al. Sleep enforces the temporal order in memory. *PLoS ONE* 2007; 2: e376.

Foulkes, D. *Children's Dreaming and the Development of Consciousness*. Cambridge, MA: Harvard University Press, 2002; ISBN 067400971.

Mullington JM, et al. Sleep loss and inflammation. *Best Practice and Research: Clinical Endocrinology and Metabolism* 2010; 24: 775–84.

National Sleep Foundation. 2004. *2004 Sleep in America Poll*.

"Sleep makes your memories stronger, and helps with creativity," *Science Daily*, November 13, 2010. *http://www.theoi.com/Daimon/Hypnos.html*.

Van Cauter E, and Knutson KL. Sleep and the epidemic of obesity in children and adults. *European Journal of Endocrinology* 2008; 159: S59–S66.

Van Dongen HPA, et al. The cumulative cost of additional wakefulness: dose-response effects on neurobehavioral functions and sleep physiology from chronic sleep restriction and total sleep deprivation. *Sleep* 2003; 2: 117–26.

Vyazovskiy VV, et al. Local sleep in awake rat. *Nature* 2011; 472: 443–47.

Chapter 2

Baddock SA, et al. Differences in infant and parent behaviors during routine bed sharing compared with cot sleeping in the home setting. *Pediatrics* 2006; 117: 1599–607.

Baddock SA, et al. Sleep arrangements and behavior of bed-sharing families in the home setting. *Pediatrics* 2007; 119: e200–207.

Ball H. Airway covering during bed-sharing. *Child: Care, Health, and Development* 2009, 35: 728–37.

Blabey MH, and Gessner BD. Infant bed-sharing practices and associated risk factors among births and infant deaths in Alaska. *Public Health Reports* 2009; 124: 527–34.

Franco P, et al. Influence of swaddling on sleep and arousal characteristics of healthy infants. *Pediatrics* 2005; 115: 1307–11.

Gessner BD, et al. The association between sudden infant death syndrome and sleep-related risk factors in Alaska. *Pediatrics* 2001; 108: 923–27.

Parmelee AH, Wenner WH, and Schulz HR. Infant sleep patterns: from birth to 16 weeks of age. *Journal of Pediatrics* 1964; 65: 576–82.

Ponsonby A, et al. Factors potentiating the risk of sudden infant death syndrome associated with the prone position. *New England Journal of Medicine* 1993; 329: 377–82.

Richardson HL, et al. Influence of swaddling experience on spontaneous arousal patterns and autonomic control in sleeping infants. *Journal of Pediatrics* 2010; 157: 85–91.

Richardson HL, et al. Minimizing the risks of sudden infant death syndrome: to swaddle or not to swaddle? *Journal of Pediatrics* 2009; 155: 475–81.

Ruys J, et al. Bed-sharing in the first four months of life: a risk factor for sudden infant death. *Acta Paediatrica* 2007; 96: 1399–1403.

Shapiro-Mendoza CK, et al. US infant mortality trends attributable to accidental suffocation and strangulation in bed from 1984 through 2004: are rates increasing. *Pediatrics* 2009; 123: 533–3.

Tappin D, Ecob R, Brook H. Bedsharing, roomsharing, and sudden infant death syndrome in Scotland: a case-control study. *Journal of Pediatrics* 2005; 147: 32–37.

Task Force on Sudden Infant Death Syndrome. The changing concept of sudden infant death syndrome. *Pediatrics* 2005; 116: 1245–55, http://pedi atrics.aappublications.org/content/116/5/1245.full.

Wilson CA, et al. Clothing and bedding and its relevance to sudden infant death syndrome: further results from the New Zealand cot death study. *Journal of Paediatrics and Child Health* 1994; 30: 506–12.

Chapter 3

Ball HL. Together or apart? A behavioural and physiological investigation of sleeping arrangements for twin infants. *Midwifery* 2007; 23: 404–12.

Barr RG, et al. Age-related incidence curve of hospitalized shaken baby syndrome cases: convergent evidence for crying as a trigger to shaking. *Child Abuse and Neglect* 2006; 30: 7–16.

Catherine N, et al. Should we do more to get the word out? Causes of, responses to, and consequences of crying and colic in popular parenting magazines. *Journal of Developmental and Behavioral Pediatrics* 2005; 26: 14–23.

Chang EF, et al. Environmental noise retards auditory cortical development. *Science* 2003; 300: 498–502.

Damato EG, and Burant C. Sleep patterns and fatigue in parents of twins. *J Obstet Gynecol Neonatal Nurs.* 2008; 37: 738–49.

http://summaries.cochrane.org/CD007202/effect-of-pacifier-use-on-dura tion-of-breastfeeding-in-full-term-infants.

http://www.hipdysplasia.org/For-Physicians/Pediatricians/default.aspx.

http://www2.aap.org/sections/scan/practicingsafety/Toolkit_Resources/ Module1/swaddling.pdf.

Pennsylvania Department of Health. *Cries to Smiles.* Harrisburg, PA: Pennsylvania Department of Health, Breastfeeding Awareness and Support Group, 2007.

Chapter 4

Bei B, et al. Subjective perception of sleep, but not its objective quality, is associated with immediate postpartum mood disturbances in healthy women. *Sleep* 2010; 33: 531–38.

Dennis CL, and Ross L. Relationships among infant sleep patterns, maternal fatigue, and development of depressive symptomatology. *Birth* 2005; 32: 187–93.

Doan T, et al. Breast-feeding increases sleep duration of new parents. *Journal of Perinatal and Neonatal Nursing* 2007; 21: 200–206.

Dørheim SK, et al. Sleep and depression in postpartum women: a population-based study. *Sleep* 2009; 32: 847–55.

Dørheim SK, et al. Subjective and objective sleep among depressed and non-depressed postnatal women. *Acta Psychiatrica Scandinavica* 2009; 119: 128–36.

Maxted AE, et al. Infant colic and maternal depression. *Infant Ment Health J.* 2005; 26: 56–68.

Montgomery-Downs HE, et al. Infant feeding methods and maternal sleep and daytime functioning. *Pediatrics* 2010; 126: e1562–68.

Pinilla T, and Birch LL. Help me make it through the night: behavioral entrainment of breast-fed infants' sleep patterns. *Pediatrics* 1993; 91: 436–44.

Chapter 5

Adler M. Promoting maternal child health by teaching parents to calm fussy infants at the Boulder, Colorado, Department of Health. Presented: CDC CityMatCH Urban MCH Leadership Conf; Aug 28, 2007; Denver, CO.

Barron JJ, et al. Proton pump inhibitor utilization patterns in infants. *J Pediatr Gastroenterol Nutr* 2007; 45: 421–27.

Chapter 6

Gaylor EE, et al. A longitudinal follow-up study of young children's sleep patterns using a developmental classification system. *Behavioral Sleep Medicine* 2005; 3(1): 44–61.

Hauck FR, et al. Infant sleeping arrangements and practices during the first year of life. *Pediatrics* 2008; 122 Suppl 2: S113–20.

Henderson JM, et al. Sleeping through the night: the consolidation of self-regulated sleep across the first year of life. *Pediatrics* 2010; 126: e1081–87.

National Sleep Foundation. 2004. *2004 Sleep in America Poll.*

Yeh ES, et al. Injuries associated with cribs, playpens, and bassinets among young children in the US, 1990–2008. *Pediatrics* 2011; 127: 479-86.

Chapter 7

Anders TF, et al. Sleeping through the night: a developmental perspective. *Pediatrics* 1992; 90: 554–60.

Chasens ER, and Braxter B. Effects of breastfeeding on sleep in infants and mothers. *Sleep* 2011; 34: Abstract Supplement 0832.

Ferber SG, et al. Massage therapy by mothers enhances the adjustment of circadian rhythms to the nocturnal period in full-term infants. *Journal of Developmental and Behavioral Pediatrics* 2002; 23: 410–15.

Mindell JA, et al. A nightly bedtime routine: impact on sleep in young children and maternal mood. *Sleep* 2009; 32: 599–606.

Paul IM, et al. Preventing obesity during infancy: a pilot study. *Obesity* 2011; 19: 353–61.

Taveras EM, et al. Short sleep duration in infancy and risk of childhood overweight. *Archives of Pediatrics and Adolescent Medicine* 2008; 162: 305–11.

Chapter 8

Gaylor EE, et al. A longitudinal follow-up study of young children's sleep patterns using a developmental classification system. *Behavioral Sleep Medicine* 2005; 3(1): 44–61.

Henderson JM, et al. Sleeping through the night: the consolidation of self-regulated sleep across the first year of life. *Pediatrics* 2010; 126: e1081–87.

Hiscock H, and Wake M. Randomised controlled trial of behavioural infant sleep intervention to improve infant sleep and maternal mood. *British Medical Journal* 2002; 324: 1062–65.

Mindell JA, et al. Behavioral treatment of bedtime problems and night wakings in infants and young children. *Sleep* 2006; 29: 1263–76.

National Sleep Foundation. 2004. *2004 Sleep in America Poll.*

Rana M, et al. Etiology of obstructive sleep apnea in infants. *Sleep* 2011; 34: Abstract Supplement 0860.

Touchette E, et al. Factors associated with fragmented sleep at night across childhood. *Archives of Pediatrics and Adolescent Medicine* 2005; 159: 242–49.

Chapter 10

Anderson SE, and Whitaker RC. Household routines and obesity in US preschool-aged children. *Pediatrics* 2010; 125: 420–28.

Bell JF, and Zimmerman FJ. Shortened nighttime sleep duration in early life and subsequent childhood obesity. *Archives of Pediatrics and Adolescent Medicine* 2010; 164: 840–45.

D'Souza AL, et al. Bunk bed–related injuries among children and adolescents treated in emergency departments in the United States, 1990–2005. *Pediatrics* 2008; 121: e1696–702.

Fan Jiang, et al. Sleep and obesity in preschool children. *Journal of Pediatrics* 2009; 154: 814–18.

Garrison MM, et al. Media use and child sleep: the impact of content, timing, and environment. *Pediatrics* 128; 2011: 29–35.

Gaylor EE, et al. A longitudinal follow-up study of young children's sleep patterns using a developmental classification system. *Behavioral Sleep Medicine* 2005; 3(1): 44–61.

National Sleep Foundation. 2004. *2004 Sleep in America Poll.*

Owens J, et al. Television-viewing habits and sleep disturbance in school children. *Pediatrics* 1999; 104: e27.

Touchette E, et al. Associations between sleep duration patterns and behavioral/cognitive functioning at school entry. *Sleep* 2007; 30: 1213–19.

Touchette E, et al. Associations between sleep duration patterns and overweight/obesity at age 6. *Sleep* 2008; 31: 1507–14.

Zadnik K, et al. Myopia and ambient night-light lighting, *Nature* 2000; 404: 143–44.

Chapter 12

Afraid and confused: understanding childhood parasomnias. *American Academy of Sleep Medicine,* July 10, 2007, http://yoursleep.aasmnet.org/article.aspx?id=495.

Elias MJ, et al. Patterns of breast-fed infants in the first 2 years of life. *Pediatrics* 1986; 77: 322–29.

Jenni OG, et al. A longitudinal study of bed sharing and sleep problems among Swiss children in the first 10 years of life. *Pediatrics* 2005; 115: 233–34.

Nguyen BH, et al. Sleep terrors in children: a prospective study of twins. *Pediatrics* 2008; 122: e1164–67.

Paul IM, et al. Effect of honey, dextromethorphan, and no treatment on nocturnal cough and sleep quality for coughing children and their parents. *Archives of Pediatrics and Adolescent Medicine* 2007; 161: 1140–46.

Paul IM, Beiler JS, King TS, Clapp ER, Vallati J, and Berlin CM, Jr. Vapor rub, petrolatum, and no treatment for children with nocturnal cough and cold symptoms. *Pediatrics* 2010; 126: 1092–99.

Touchette E, et al. Factors associated with fragmented sleep at night across childhood. *Archives of Pediatrics and Adolescent Medicine* 2005; 159: 242–49.

Stampler L. Co-sleeping bad for kids? These parents kept it secret. *Huffington Post,* August 18, 2011, http://www.huffingtonpost.com/2011/08/16/closeted-co-sleepers-stig_n_928565.html.

Chapter 14

Iglowstein I, et al. Sleep duration from infancy to adolescence: reference values and generational trends. *Pediatrics* 2003; 111: 302–7.

Lam JC, et al. The effects of napping on cognitive function in preschoolers. *Journal of Developmental and Behavioral Pediatrics* 2011; 32: 90–97.

National Sleep Foundation. 2004. *2004 Sleep in America Poll.*

Weissbluth, M. Naps in children: 6 months–7 years. *Sleep* 1995; 18: 82–87.

Chapter 15

Bhattacharjee R, et al. Adenotonsillectomy outcomes in treatment of obstructive sleep apnea in children: a multicenter retrospective study. *American Journal of Respiratory and Critical Care Medicine* 2010; 182: 676–83.

Brain basics: understanding sleep. National Institute of Neurological Disorders and Stroke, http://www.ninds.nih.gov/disorders/brain_basics/understanding_sleep.htm#Tips.

Goldman S, et al. Behavior and sleep—associations across childhood and adolescence in autism spectrum disorder. Presentation to the International Society for Autism Research (INSAR), May 12, 2011.

Jan JE, et al. Sleep hygiene for children with neurodevelopmental disabilities. *Pediatrics* 2008; 122: 1343–50.

Jan JE, et al. Use of melatonin in the treatment of paediatric sleep disorders. *Journal of Pineal Research* 2007; 21: 193–9.

Li AM, et al. Prevalence and risk factors of habitual snoring in primary school children. *Chest* 2010; 138: 519–27.

Stojanovski SD, et al. Trends in medication prescribing for pediatric sleep difficulties in US outpatient settings. *Sleep* 2007; 30: 1013–17.

Resources

SIDS

American SIDS Institute
Phone: (800) 232-7437
www.SIDS.org
First Candle/SIDS Alliance
www.firstcandle.org
Sudden Infant Death Syndrome Network
www.sids-network.org

Snoring, Apnea, and Sleep Disordered Breathing

American Sleep Apnea Association
www.sleepapnea.org
National Institutes of Health
http://www.ninds.nih.gov/disor ders/sleep_apnea/sleep_apnea .htm
National Center on Sleep Disorders Research
www.nhlbi.nih.gov/about/ncsdr/ index.htm
Night Terrors Resource Center
www.nightterrors.org

Breastfeeding

U.S. Department of Health
www.womenshealth.gov/ breastfeeding/
La Leche League
www.llli.org

Crib Safety

Consumer Reports
www.consumerreports.org
U.S. Consumer Product Safety Commission
Phone: (800) 638-2772
www.cpsc.org

National Safety Council
www.nsc.org

General Sleep Information

American Academy of Pediatrics
www.aap.org
www.healthychildren.org
American Academy of Sleep Medicine
www.sleepeducation.com
American Academy of Sleep Medicine
http://www.aasmnet.org
BabyCenter.com
www.babycenter.com/expert/ faq-babysleep.htm
www.babycenter.com/expert/ faq-toddlersleep.htm
National Sleep Foundation
www.sleepfoundation.org
Sleepnet
www.sleepnet.com
Zero to Three
www.zerotothree.org

Other Resources

Postpartum Support International (Postpartum Depression)
www.postpartum.net
National Organization of Mothers of Twins Clubs
www.nomotc.org
March of Dimes (Parents of Premature Babies)
www.marchofdimes.com

Index

cry it out (CIO) (*continued*)
  three to five months, 126–27
  toddlers/preschoolers, 254–57, 259–61
cuddlies. *See* loveys
cuddling, 44, 144–45, 244

D

dads
  calming babies, 87
  partner relationship tips, 110–11
  putting toddlers/preschoolers to sleep, 299–300
daily diary. *See* diaries
daily routines. *See also* bedtime routines
  children's love of, 130, 209–10
Damato, Elizabeth, 93–94
David, Laurie, 225
Daylight Savings Time, 252–54
day-night confusion, of newborns, 121
day/night cycle, 9, 15–17. *See also* circadian rhythm
daytime feeding, 101, 175–76, 266
daytime sleeping, 135, 219
deep breathing. *See* magic breathing
deep ("slow wave") sleep, 18, 20
dehumidifiers, 320
depression. *See* postpartum depression

developmental problems, 328–30. *See also* autism
diaper rashes, 105
diaries, 153–54, 159, 229–30
  sample, 339
diarrhea, 105
diet. *See* bottle-feeding; breast-feeding; feedings
dimming the lights, 242, 283, 298, 330
Dinges, David, 13
distractions
  mealtime, 175, 198, 266
  napping and, 309, 312, 313
  waking at night, 165–70
  white noise for. *See* white noise
disturbances. *See* sleep problems
doll (or puppet) play, 238–39, 274, 299
dopamine, 14
"Dr. No," 208, 234–35
dream feeds, 39, 101, 168–70
  defined, 343
dreams, 22, 25–26. *See also* bad dreams
drippy noses, 319–20
drowsiness, 19, 20, 167
drunk vs. sleep deprived, 13
dry throat, 267–68
DUDU wrap, 69–71

E

early bedtimes, 158, 182, 285, 286

early morning light, 62, 119–20
early waking, 183–84, 285–88
easy-going (calm) temperament, 33, 35, 205, 261
"eat, play, sleep" sequence, 90–91
eating. *See* bottle-feeding; breast-feeding; feedings
Emerson, Ralph Waldo, 142
endorphins, 82
exercises
  for PPD, 116
  tummy, 54, 55–56
extinction, 185–86
  graduated, 186–90
extinction bursts, 190, 260–61
eye masks, 109, 338

F

face covering, and bed-sharing, 49–50
fading. *See* pick up/put down
fairy tales, 239–40, 246, 274
  defined, 343
family beds. *See* bed-sharing
Family Dinner, The (David), 225
family meetings, 217, 249–51
  defined, 343
Fast-Food Rule, 211, 231, 237
  defined, 343
fathers. *See* dads
fatigue. *See* tiredness

reading. *See* Beddy-Bye book; book reading

red alerts. *See* medical issues

reflexes, 37, 64. *See also* calming reflex

REM sleep, 18–19, 19, 21–22
defined, 344
at different ages, 24–25

resistant children. *See* spirited temperament

resources, 354

retraining, helping infants after they backslide, 194

reverse psychology to boost pacifier use, 83–84, 98
defined, 344

rhythmic behavior. *See* rocking; swinging

rice cereal, 4, 133

right-brain Happiest Toddler communication. *See* gossiping; magic breathing; patience-stretching; Toddler-ese

right-brain language, 212–13

rigidity, 208–9, 329

rocking, 77–78, 131, 296–97. *See also* swinging
head banging and, 172–73
myths about, 40

role-playing, 273–74
defined, 344–45

rolling over, 49, 55–56, 57, 69–70, 71

room sharing, 138–39. *See also* bed-sharing

room temperature, 51

roughhousing, 154, 235, 241, 298, 329

routines. *See also* bedtime routines
children's love of, 130, 209–10

rubber nipples, 82

runny noises, 319–20

S

SAD (seasonal affective disorder), 116, 335

saline spray, 268

Salk, Lee, 41

schedules. *See* sleep schedules

science of sleep, 6–28
children vs. adults, 22–26
circadian rhythm, 15–17
myths about sleep, 7–9
REM and NREM sleep, 18–22
sleep deprivation, 11–12

Scientist in the Crib (Gopnik, Meltzoff and Kuhl), 129

SDB. *See* sleep-disordered breathing

seasonal affective disorder (SAD), 116, 335

seizures, nighttime, 327–28

self-soothing, 39, 40, 70, 85, 166

sensitive temperament, 34, 101, 128, 138, 187, 311

separation anxiety, 271–75, 277

setting goals, 160

shaken baby syndrome (SBS), 80–81

shaking babies, 80–81

Sharkey, Kathryn, 333

shivers, 68–69

short phrases, 212–13

shushing, 71–77. *See also* white noise
loudness of different sounds, 72
myths about, 75–76
secrets for successful, 72–73

side-door lessons, 216, 238–40
defined, 345

side/stomach position, 71, 146

SIDS (sudden infant death syndrome), 52–55
bed-sharing and, 49–50, 54
common ages, 53
protecting against, 53–54, 82–83
resources, 354
swaddling and, 56–58

sign language, 207

silicone pacifiers, 82

sinus infections, 319–20

sitting down, 199–200

skin rashes, 105, 118

skipping naps, 315–16

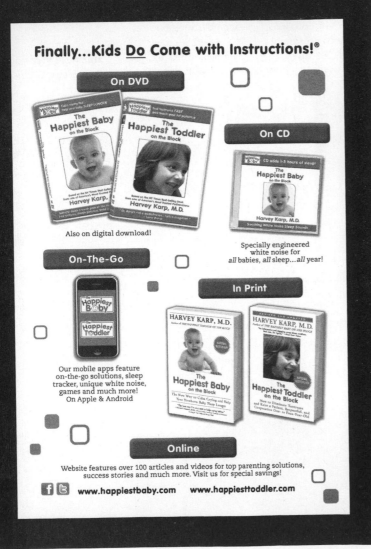

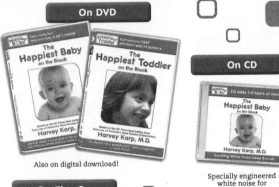
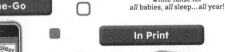
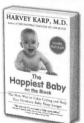
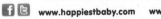